ALSO BY JANICE COX

Natural Beauty at Home
Natural Beauty for All Seasons

Natural Beauty from the Garden

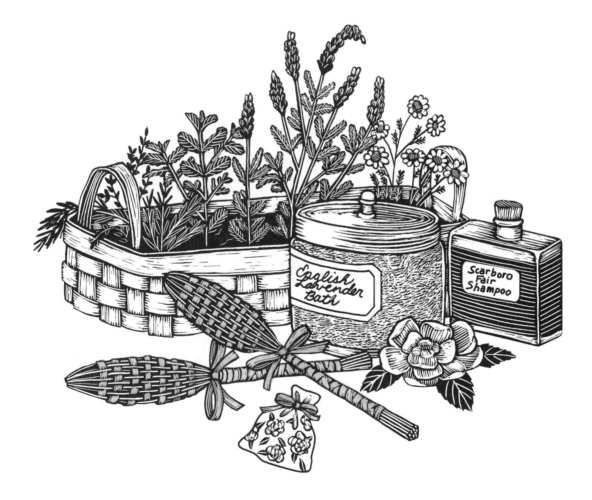

Natural Beauty from the Garden

MORE THAN 200 DO-IT-YOURSELF BEAUTY RECIPES AND GARDEN IDEAS

Janice Cox

Illustrated by Dorothy Reinhardt

An Owl Book

Henry Holt and Company
New York

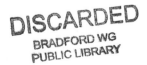

Henry Holt and Company, Inc.
Publishers since 1866
115 West 18th Street
New York, New York 10011

Henry Holt® is a registered trademark
of Henry Holt and Company, Inc.

Published in Canada by Fitzhenry & Whiteside Ltd.,
195 Allstate Parkway, Markham, Ontario L3R 4T8.

Library of Congress Cataloging-in-Publication Data
Cox, Janice.
Natural beauty from the garden: more than 200 do-it-yourself
beauty recipes and garden ideas / Janice Cox.
p.   cm.
"An Owl book."
Includes index.
ISBN 0-8050-5781-1 (pbk.: alk. paper)
1. Beauty, Personal.   2. Herbal cosmetics.   3. Skin—Care and hygiene.
4. Hair—Care and hygiene.   5. Toilet preparations.   6. Gardening—
Therapeutic use.   I. Title.
RA778.C757   1999   98-19042
646.72—dc21   CIP

Henry Holt books are available for special promotions and
premiums. For details contact: Director, Special Markets.

First Edition 1999

DESIGNED BY LUCY ALBANESE

Printed in the United States of America
All first editions are printed on acid-free paper. ∞
1   3   5   7   9   10   8   6   4   2

To my parents who have always
encouraged me to grow!
And to my wonderful husband, Ray,
and our two beautiful daughters,
Lauren and Marie —

Thank you for a life full of
happiness, beauty, and flowers!

Acknowledgments

Creating a book is very similar to creating a garden. It requires thought, design, study, and a bit of weeding. I am extremely fortunate to have worked with a talented group of individuals on this project. They all were an invaluable part of my "beauty garden team."

To all of my dear friends, family members, and readers: Thank you for your ideas, advice, and kind letters of support.

To my agent, Laurie Harper: Thank you for your seeds of literary wisdom and insight. Your enthusiasm always gives me a boost.

To my editor at Henry Holt and Company, Amelia Sheldon: Thank you for your direction, advice, and positive attitude. You are a delight to work with; I look forward to your phone calls.

To Wendy Sherman, Vice President at Owl Books: Thank you for your support. This is our third book together and I cannot thank you enough for sharing my vision of natural beauty.

Special thank-yous to Raquel Jaramillo for her beautiful cover design, Lucy Albanese for the overall book design, Dorothy Reinhardt for her stunning artwork, and Erin Clermont for her very thorough job of copy editing. You are all the best.

A final thank-you to everyone at Henry Holt and Company for your efforts in making my job pure pleasure.

When you plant a garden, you plant beauty. Keep growing, you are all beautiful!

Note

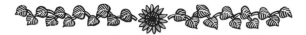

Contents

Facial Care Products and Treatments............................ *71*

Body Care Products and Treatments.............................*209*

Massage and Relaxation *233*

Welcome to My Garden!

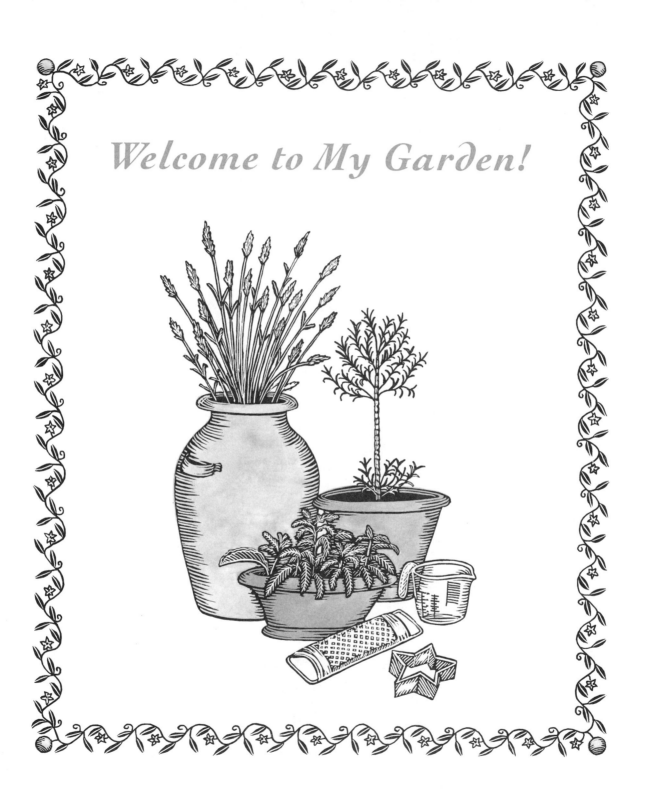

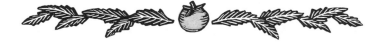

*O*ne day I went out to my garden to harvest a few vegetables, gather some herbs, and do some weeding. It was there, among all my growing plants, that I came up with the idea for this book. I thought of all the wonderful products and treatments that this small corner of my yard provided—natural beauty from the garden!—and this book was born. I have written two other books on home beauty: *Natural Beauty at Home* and *Natural Beauty for All Seasons*. Together they contain over 400 recipes for making your own natural cosmetic products. After I finished those, however, I still had several recipes and ideas for beauty treatments that I wanted to share. But I had been struggling with the right presentation. Now, I had it.

My first book, *Natural Beauty at Home*, came together quite quickly. I was so excited to share the wonderful world of home beauty that I simply chose my favorite recipes from those I had been gathering and perfecting over the years. *Natural Beauty for All Seasons* became an obvious follow-up when I noticed how many of my friends and readers were giving their products as gifts and using fresh seasonal ingredients. So a book on year-round beauty and gift-giving ideas made total sense. But a third book, containing even more natural beauty recipes? Was it possible? Yes, and this is it. I think this one is my best project to date!

My other books came from my kitchen. This one originated in my garden. Once the seed of the idea had been planted I went inside and began compiling various botanical recipes, garden designs, planting tips, projects, and new spa treatments. I got out all my notes from garden club talks I had given, magazine articles I had written, and reader letters I received containing gardening tips and stories. The book began to grow rapidly, its contents covering my antique rolltop desk, where I do all of my writing. Now I see what a natural this concept was—after all, what better place to find beauty than outside, in the garden?

I am pleased to continue sharing natural, homemade beauty recipes in this series of books. Creating my own treatments and cosmetics has been an activity that has given me pleasure for years. I started making my own beauty products at a very young age. My father was a farmer, which meant we lived in the country. Commercial beauty products were hard to buy because they were sold in town and I was too young to drive. I loved reading beauty books and magazines for hours in my room; they gave me ideas. I spent even more hours in our family bathroom mixing up my own potions, lotions, and treatments. My grandmother was my inspiration. She is a beautiful woman who has always enjoyed her own homemade beauty products and treatments. A visit to her house was always special. The first time I had a real manicure or placed cotton pads soaked in witch hazel over my eyes was in her home. Today she is in her nineties and is still my best beauty advisor. Little did I know that those happy times with her would turn into the lifelong project of learning, sharing, and discovering that it has for me.

If you have read my other books, then you are already familiar with how wonderful my recipes are. If, on the other hand, this is your first time—welcome! This book combines my two favorite activities—home beauty and gardening. I hope you will enjoy using it as much as I enjoyed creating it. Working in my garden with plants, flowers, and herbs made writing this book a sheer delight. I hope it inspires you to go out into your own yard and see it in a new and different light. Even if you have never gardened before, you can plant a few bath herbs for your home or start a small skin-care garden, which I will give you pointers on starting. Whether you live in the country or a big city, don't feel limited by space or the fact that you may not be an expert gardener. Everyone can grow a natural beauty garden that suits their personal needs and resources!

Of course, I do not expect you to plant every ingredient necessary for creating the recipes in this book. In fact, all of the fresh ingredients here can easily be found at grocery stores, farmers' markets, or natural food stores. If you are inclined to look, you may even find some of the ingredients growing in your neighborhood or in nearby fields. I have found several plants, such as dandelions, clover, chickweed, and poppies, in these spots. You may also want to exchange a few plants with a friend or neighbor and share the different recipes you've made. Just remember to be careful when picking in areas other than your own yard. Check that the plants you gather have not been sprayed with any harmful chemicals and be sure to have the property owner's permission if you venture onto another's land.

This book contains more than 200 simple, easy-to-make recipes for your body, bath, and hair, as well as some additional tips and features I thought you'd enjoy. The recipes are organized by how they are used—from head to toe. I have also included a few special sections, such as children's bath ideas and fragrance products. There are garden projects and designs for outdoor showers, container gardens, and even directions for growing a cucumber inside a bottle! Instructions for many of my family's favorite herbal crafts, such as lavender wands, flower hat bands, and potpourri blends are here for your enjoyment as well. Throughout the book you'll see I have sprinkled Garden Notes. These are brief and simple green-thumb tips and trivia I have picked up over the years. All in all, I like to think of the contents of this book as the perfect combination of cooking and handicraft, which anyone can master.

Once you've made your first cosmetic product I'm convinced that, just like me, you'll be hooked on whipping up a continual and growing variety of them. After all, who can resist the world of natural beauty; it is fun, creative, and healthy. After using many of your own natural products and treatments, the added benefit will be how terrific you look and feel.

The recipes in this book are easy to follow and use common ingredients. I believe that if you can read a recipe you can create your own products. This is certainly true with my recipes. Many of the procedures involve simply mixing together a few ingredients in the right proportions and pouring them into a clean container. There is no need for expensive equipment; common kitchen items are all that you will need.

In addition to the satisfaction you will receive from making and using your own products, the cost savings are also attractive. When you realize what you have been spending on commercial products (a majority of the price is based on packaging and advertising, not the cost of the actual ingredients), you will be delighted at the low cost of your own products and treatments. In a fancy bath boutique I recently saw a gorgeous wine bottle filled with herbal bath salts for $25. I made those same salts for less than $2 in ingredients and recycled my own bottle! (See pages 201–3 for recipes.)

I hope this book gives you the opportunity to try something new, celebrate yourself, and really feel good from head to toe. There is an old folk saying that ends, "If you want to be happy forever, become a gardener." I couldn't agree more. I would add, though, if you want to be happy and beautiful, take what you can from the garden and incorporate it into your bath and beauty regime.

Let's get started!

TEN STEPS TO NATURAL BEAUTY

1. Get plenty of rest.
2. Exercise regularly.
3. Eat a balanced diet.
4. Take breaks to boost your energy—meditate, walk, or just relax.
5. Keep your skin and hair clean and full of moisture.
6. Use sun protection.
7. Brush and floss your teeth regularly.
8. Drink plenty of water—at least eight glasses a day.
9. Give yourself a monthly body treatment head to toe.
10. Use natural beauty products.

Making your own cosmetic products is not a new concept; women have been doing it for centuries. We have all heard of Cleopatra's legendary milk baths, or Puritan women and their homemade lipsticks. Throughout history great beauties have always made their own special treatments, it seems. After all, not so long ago, homemade versions were all people had to use. Today, it's the opposite. There are more bath and beauty products available on store shelves than anyone could possibly use. Cosmetics featuring natural products is now one of the fastest growing areas of the beauty industry. When I began writing about home beauty, these naturally inspired products were somewhat hard to find. I define as "natural" those products that do not contain any manmade materials. They are as nature created them, pure and unpreserved. Today, soaps, bath salts, and essential oils with labels touting natural ingredients are sold even at my local grocery store. I like to compare this growing phenomenon of enhancing natural products to recycling. I remember it used to be quite difficult to recycle your paper, glass, or plastic. You had to seek out recycling centers. Now, in many towns you can simply set your items out on the curb, have them taken away by a local disposal company, and delivered to community recycling centers. Similarly, terms like "aromatherapy," "hydrotherapy," and "meditation" were embraced by a small group of people. Currently, they are a part of our vocabulary and becoming a part of our everyday life. Both of these changes and many others reflect our growing consciousness of the earth's offerings and the importance of using and preserving them wisely. Many people have found this new attitude adds to the fulfillment they feel.

Simplification has also become a lifestyle choice, and getting back to basics is a very vogue thing to do. I love it that I am finally "in style." I have always enjoyed homemade items. I make my own beauty products because they are safe, convenient, fun, and also save money, along with being an extremely relaxing and creative activity. I think homemade cosmetic products are a wonderful addition to anyone's lifestyle; they are a unique blend of cooking, craft, gardening, and nature. Making them also includes a focus on looking and·feeling your best and taking good care of yourself. This natural enhancement of ourselves is something we should all strive to include in our activities each day.

Many of my readers express their concerns about commercial product additives, asking, Are they really necessary? Yes. Commercial products are created in huge batches and must have very long shelf lives and be able to withstand temperature changes during shipping and storage before being sold. In fact, I would not purchase a product that did not have some sort of preservative, ensuring its safety and freshness. Now, with home beauty, this is no longer necessary. As the manufacturer of your own products you can make a fresh product before each use, or simply throw it out and mix up a new batch if one goes bad. The former option is especially helpful for onetime treatments such as facial masks, hair-conditioning packs, and special baths.

Convenience is another added bonus to home beauty. If it is late at night or early in the morning and you are in the mood for a bit of pampering, you probably have the makings for several products right in your own home. There is no need to go to the store or book an appointment at your local spa. Whip up a fresh facial mask or give yourself a total pedicure whenever you wish. I know this is especially helpful for new mothers. They definitely can use some extra attention and pampering. Natural, at-home beauty routines fit into the newborn's schedule which often makes it hard for mothers to leave the house.

The recipes in this book do not contain any artificial colors or fragrance. Indeed, many can be made fragrance-free. You'll see that in many recipes I have suggested different scents, but these are always optional ingredients. The normal color and scent of my products is derived from their own natural ingredients. These look and smell wonderful on their own, as nature intended!

Preservatives are not needed for most of these recipes because certain ingredients included in them, such as vitamin E, vitamin C, and tincture of benzoin, act as natural preservatives. If you choose not to use a preservative that's been suggested, you may need to refrigerate the product in order to maintain its freshness.

If you are sensitive to a known ingredient, say, olive oil, either find a suitable substitution, such as almond oil, or choose a different recipe to make. You should know that you can be sensitive to natural beauty products just as you can to commercial products. If you have a known food allergy, such as to tomatoes, chances are you will also be allergic to cosmetic products that contain tomatoes, even though you're not ingesting them. Just to be safe, take special care when using a new product or treatment. Always spot-test it first: Apply a small amount of the new product to the skin on the inside of your arm and wait twenty-four hours. If there is no reaction, it is probably safe to proceed with the treatment. If you have extremely sensitive skin or have a long list of allergies, it is always best to consult a dermatologist or physician before using any new product or treatment.

Remember, you are the manufacturer of these cosmetic products and quality control is therefore *your* responsibility. Always work with clean equipment and pure ingredients. If you are purchasing fresh or dried ingredients, it is important that they are meant for human consumption rather than decorative purposes. Some dried flowers intended for decoration contain harmful dyes and preservatives that could find their way into your cosmetics. You are usually safe using ingredients that can be ingested.

The following is a list of basic care and storage guidelines to ensure a long and healthy shelf life for your homemade cosmetic products:

1. Always store your products in the cleanest of jars and bottles.

2. Keep your fingers out of the container as much as possible. Always wash your hands before handling cosmetics. Remember, each time you dip your fingers into the containers, you introduce foreign germs and materials to the mix. Try to use cotton balls, cotton swabs, or a small spatula when possible, or *pour* your products onto clean hands.

3. Store your products in a cool, dark, dry place. Heat and light can sometimes alter their composition.

4. If the ingredients in a product separate, don't worry. Simply stir the mixture thoroughly or re-blend, using a hand mixer or a blender.

5. If something smells bad or changes color, it is best to throw it out. Once a product has gone bad there is no way to recover it; it's best to just make a new batch.

Below is a list of tools you will need for making the cosmetics and beauty treatments in this book. Many are common kitchen items that you already own. You will probably not need all of the items listed. For example, a blender, electric mixer, and a spoon can all be used for stirring. Always remember to keep your equipment clean; you don't want to introduce foreign ingredients into your cosmetic products and onto your body.

Grater: I like to use a standard handheld metal cheese grater for beeswax, soap, and vegetables.

Vegetable peeler: I use this for peeling vegetables and grating beeswax and soap. I prefer to use a vegetable peeler for grating beeswax and cocoa butter, since it is faster and easier to clean.

Citrus peeler and zester: This tool is handy for peeling citrus fruits and removing the "zest" or colored part of the peel. This is not essential, but it's a fun gadget to have. You can do just as well using a sharp paring knife.

Measuring cups and spoons: These are a must for measuring ingredients correctly.

Glass ovenproof measuring cups with pouring spouts: I use these for everything. They can be put in a hot water bath on the stove, in the microwave, and in the refrigerator. Glass will not react with any of your cosmetic ingredients and is easy to clean.

Stirring rod: I use a chopstick as a stirring rod. It isn't essential, but it makes stirring small amounts easy. It also makes me feel like more of a cosmetic chemist.

Pans: Steel and enamel pans work best. Aluminum and iron sometimes react with ingredients, especially when you are making soap.

Microwave: This is not entirely necessary, but it really speeds things up when it comes to heating and melting times.

Blender and/or food processor: These tools are perfect for really mixing up creams and lotions. You can stir pretty well by hand, but a blender makes the task so much easier and faster. Make sure your blender is dishwasher-safe to cut down on cleaning time.

Juicer: This is a handy appliance that can be used for creating fresh juices from herbs, vegetables, and fruits.

Hand mixer or electric whisk: Both speed up mixing of creams and lotions as a blender does, but because they are handheld you have a little more direct control.

Coffee or spice grinder: Use these for grinding peels and herbs. Make sure you clean your coffee grinder well after each use or your coffee may taste a bit funny. Spice grinders and small food processors also work well for these tasks.

Funnel: This item is essential for bottling your products and filtering solutions.

Coffee filters, cheesecloth, paper towels: All can be used as filtering material, placed inside funnels and strainers before solutions and mixtures are poured through.

Knives: You need some sharp ones for cutting and chopping.

Glass and ceramic bowls: These are ideal for mixing, heating in the microwave, and storing products.

Eyedropper: A handy item for adding scents and natural preservatives.

Strainer: This is a must-have for straining solutions and mixtures. Tea strainers work especially well and fit most small jars.

Old muffin tins, loaf pans, cookie cutters, and small cardboard boxes: Use these for molds when making soap.

Stove top, warming plate, or electric skillet: You will need heat to melt ingredients in some of the recipes. If you do not have a stove available, you can use an electric skillet with one to two inches of water to create a water bath that will provide all the heat necessary for creating most of these beauty items.

Assorted jars, bottles, bowls, and spray bottles: You will want to have a number of these handy for storing and applying your cosmetics. These containers can be found in a variety of places: grocery stores, drugstores, department stores, and stores specializing in cooking equipment. Put your recycling creativity to use as well. Before you throw out an old jar, bottle, or container, think of how it could be reused for your own cosmetics products. Plastic honey bears and sport-drink squeeze bottles are great for lotions, shampoos, and liquid soaps. Wine and liquor bottles are perfect for scented oils and bath mixtures. Even your old commercial cosmetic containers can be used to hold your new homemade versions.

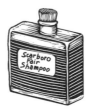

WEIGHTS AND MEASURES

3 teaspoons = 1 tablespoon

4 tablespoons = ¼ cup

8 tablespoons = ½ cup

12 tablespoons = ¾ cup

16 tablespoons = 1 cup

2 tablespoons = 1 ounce

1 cup = 8 ounces

1 cup = ½ pint

2 cups = 1 pint

4 cups = 1 quart

4 quarts = 1 gallon

juice of 1 lemon = about 3 tablespoons

juice of 1 orange = about ⅓ cup

METRIC EQUIVALENTS

1 ounce = 28.35 grams

1 gram = 0.035 ounce

1 quart = 0.946 liter

1 liter = 1.06 quarts

Basic Household Ingredients

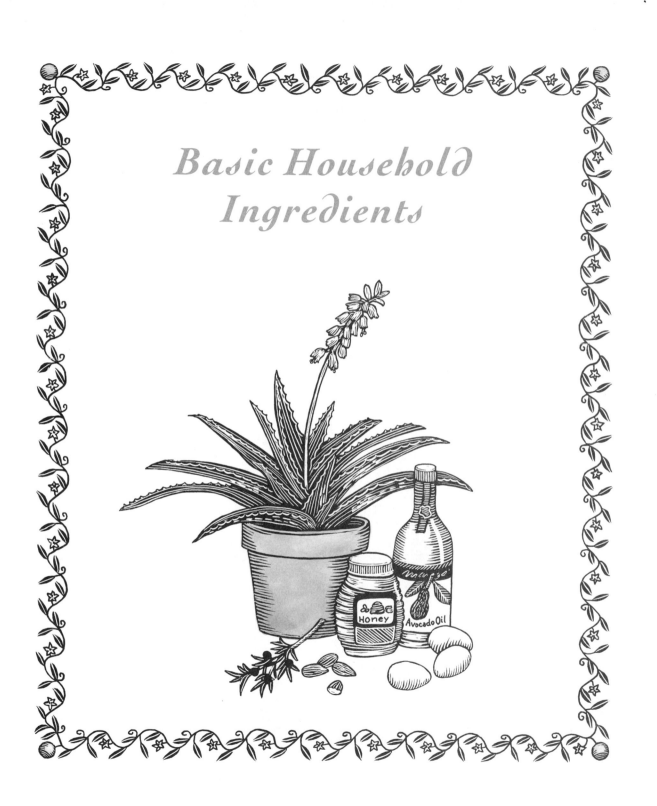

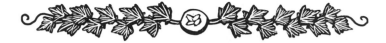

*T*he recipes in this book are inspired by the garden — the main ingredients come from plants. It is almost impossible, however, to create natural cosmetic products without several household ingredients. Many commercial products also contain these common basics. Although you may feel you need a degree in chemistry to interpret some of the ingredients listed, many of them are known to us by more familiar names. Substances such as ascorbic acid (vitamin C), tocopherol (vitamin E), *Hamamelis virginiana* (witch hazel), and *Ricinus communis* (castor oil) can all be found on product labels. I once saw a bath-soak product in a department store whose label read: "Sodium Chloride and Sodium Bicarbonate." More simply, the twenty-dollar jar of unscented minerals was made of common table salt and baking soda!

These common household ingredients are used to preserve, add texture, and blend the botanical components of each recipe. They enhance the effectiveness of the natural cosmetic products the organic items produce. You probably already have many of them in your kitchen pantry or in your bathroom cabinet that make wonderful cosmetic products on their own. For example, canola oil can be used as a makeup remover, oatmeal makes a wonderful skin cleanser, honey an excellent hair conditioner, and fresh eggs a classic skin beautifier when used as a simple facial mask.

You can usually find these household ingredients at your local grocery or pharmacy. For some ingredients, such as beeswax or essential oils, you may want to check with a good natural foods store. The shopping resources available in your area will determine the extent of your search. I can purchase coconut oil at my local grocery store, but friends had to go to a natural food store to find it. Farmers' markets and herb farms are also wonderful sources of fresh and dried ingredients.

What follows is not a complete list of all the ingredients you'll need, just the primary ones. I have also included information about ingredients in the introduction to some of the individual recipes and treatments.

Alcohol: Isopropyl alcohol (rubbing alcohol) vapors can make some people dizzy and sick to their stomachs. Therefore, I like to use natural alcohols such as vodka, gin, and rum in my products. Vodka is probably the one I use the most in my recipes because it is gentle, virtually fragrance free, and colorless. It is a natural alcohol made from grains and works well, so take advantage of the cost savings it provides. Vodka made in the United States is ethyl alcohol (ethanol) and water. The percentage of ethanol is one half the proof; for example, a 90 proof vodka is 45 percent ethanol. Gin made from juniper berries and rum made from molasses also enhance many recipes. You can buy these at your local liquor shop or, depending on the laws in your state, in the grocery store.

Baking soda: Baking soda is a gentle alkaline white powder that neutralizes acids. When mixed with acids such as vinegar, carbon dioxide is produced. This common household product has dozens of beauty applications. It can be used as a skin soother in the bath, a tooth powder, and a deodorizer when mixed with body powders. It also makes a cleansing hair rinse that no commercial product compares to for getting your hair super clean and removing residues left from styling products. Many stylists suggest a baking soda rinse before coloring or using permanent wave solutions on your hair for this reason. Baking soda can be purchased at any grocery store.

Beeswax: Beeswax, a substance secreted from the underside of bees, is the material bees use to make the walls of the honeycomb. We have yet to create a synthetic product with all of its properties. Beeswax is a valued ingredient in the cosmetics industry because its high levels of potassium prevent it from becoming rancid. It also has wonderful germ-killing properties. In beauty products it forms a protective barrier on the skin to guard against environmental irritants and lock in moisture. I buy my beeswax from a local beekeeper who sells honey at the farmers' market. You can also find it at many natural food stores and beekeeping supply shops (check your Yellow Pages under "Beekeeping").

Borax: Borax is a natural chemical substance found on alkaline lake shores. It is used as a water softener, preservative, and texturizer. Because it is a mild alkali, borax gently cleanses without drying the skin. In cream and lotion recipes it acts as an emulsifier, keeping the oils and water mixed together. Borax powder can be found in the detergent section of the grocery store.

Cocoa butter: Cocoa butter is a creamy, fatty wax that is solid at room temperature. It is obtained from the seeds of the cocoa plant. Chocolate lovers will enjoy cocoa butter's mild chocolate scent. An excellent skin softener, it can be used alone or mixed with other ingredients. Many pregnant women use it on their stomachs to avoid stretch marks. You can find cocoa butter in any drugstore—just be sure to look for products that contain 100 percent cocoa butter. I like to buy it in a solid stick, which makes it easy to rub on to your skin and lips.

Cornstarch: Cornstarch is a fine white starchy powder made from corn. Sometimes you will see it sold as "corn flour." It soothes the skin and is believed to possess healing properties. Many people use cornstarch in place of talcum powder to stay dry and fresh feeling. It also makes a good thickening agent for creams and lotions. I normally find it at the grocery store in the baking section.

Dairy products: Milk, cream, yogurt, and sour cream are all high in protein, calcium, and vitamins, and make soothing cleansers. They also contain lactose, an alpha hydroxy acid that gently sloughs off dead cells, leaving your skin soft and smooth. Milk baths were made popular by the Egyptian queen Cleopatra, who was known for her incomparable beauty. It is important to rinse well after using dairy products, as the milk could spoil if left on your skin. Dairy products are easily found at all grocery stores and markets.

Eggs: Eggs are rich in protein and make good skin and hair conditioners. Egg yolks are rich in lecithin, a natural emollient. Egg whites are naturally astringent, which means they help shrink or tighten your skin's pores. A gentle shampoo can be made simply by using a raw egg to clean your hair. Rinse well with cool water (hot water may cook the egg). Because eggs are inexpensive and easy to find, they are one of the most popular at-home beauty ingredients. Eggs are also a grocery store staple.

Epsom salts: Epsom salts, also known as magnesium sulfate, is a fine white crystal powder that you can purchase in any drugstore. The salts' name comes from where they were first discovered, at a mineral spring in Epsom, England. These natural salts are a key ingredient in many bath salt products. Soaking in them is soothing to sore muscles because they are mildly astringent. They increase your circulation and help warm tired muscles. Some people also take these salts for indigestion. Epsom salts can be found in any drugstore.

Essential oils: Essential oils are highly concentrated, aromatic extracts of different plants. They come in a wide variety of scents ranging from common ones, such as peppermint, to the more exotic patchouli and sandalwood. They are more expensive than other scents, but worth it because the scents are pure, intense, and will last for a very long time. You only need a drop or two to scent most recipes. I purchase these fragrant oils at health food stores or aromatherapy shops.

Glycerine: Glycerine is a clear, odorless, sticky liquid produced during soap making. It attracts moisture and keeps products from drying out. You will notice it listed on the ingredient labels of many cosmetic products. A classic hand softening formula is glycerine and rosewater. I purchase glycerine at the grocery store in the health care section; pharmacies also often carry it.

Honey: Honey contains many vital vitamins and minerals and is made by bees from the nectar of flowering plants and trees. It has a very high potassium content, which is why it is almost impossible for bacteria to survive in it. Honey is one of the best-known humectants, which are materials that hold moisture. My favorite way to use honey is in the bath: Adding a tablespoon or two to the tub makes your skin feel like silk! Honey is available in grocery and natural food stores. There are many different varieties, such as clover or sage, based on what blossoms the bees find near their hive.

Natural oils: Pure natural oils are excellent for moisturizing the skin and hair. They are the main ingredients for my cream and lotion recipes. I also like to use natural oils in bath products, lip balms, and massage oils. Some of my favorites are avocado, sesame, sunflower, almond, walnut, and olive oil, all of which can easily be found at your local grocery store. There are also several tropical oils, such as coconut, macadamia, and kukui nut oils, that you can find in specialty food shops or through mail-order sources. Jojoba bean oil, which is used in several recipes here, is made from the jojoba plant and is more of a plant wax than an oil.

Nuts: Almonds, walnuts, and hazelnuts all grow on trees and are usually harvested in the fall. They are rich in natural oils and make effective skin exfoliators when ground and added to cleansers and body scrubs. Their expressed oils are the basis for numerous natural creams and lotions. Nuts can be found at your local grocery store or gourmet food shop year-round. I also watch the classified section of our local paper in which many growers will advertise fresh nuts for sale. These farms are also a good source of nut hulls, which can be used in making darkening hair dyes.

Oatmeal: Oatmeal is a popular breakfast cereal that is rich in protein, potassium, iron, phosphates, magnesium, and silicon. It has gentle cleansing properties and can be used in place of soap. Oatmeal is nontoxic and soothing to the skin, so it's especially good for sensitive skin. The more inexpensive full-grain oatmeal (not quick-cooking) works best when you are making cosmetic products. It is found in the cereal section at the grocery store.

Salt: Salt is in every kitchen cupboard. You can use it as an astringent and antiseptic in cosmetics. Salt can also be used for removing dead skin from the body and scalp. I would not suggest using salt on your face or irritated skin, as it can be very drying.

Vinegar: When fruit juice ferments it turns into vinegar. Vinegars are known for their high acid content and sharp odors. In cosmetics, vinegar is used to neutralize alkaline residues left on your skin and hair. These residues are left over from the use of soap and other cleansing products. Our bodies have a natural acid level that is helpful in combating bacteria. Vinegar helps restore this healthy level. *Never apply straight vinegar to your body.* Instead, dilute the vinegar with clean water (one part vinegar to eight parts water) and rinse. Vinegar can be purchased at the grocery store.

Vitamins: Vitamins and vitamin oils are added to cosmetic products mainly for their preservative properties. Vitamins A, C, and E will all extend your recipe's shelf life and keep it from spoiling. They also have many skin-beautifying properties. Vitamins A and E oils have been used for years to moisturize and heal the skin. Vitamin C is being added to many commercial products for its antioxidant properties and is believed to give the skin a more youthful appearance. I use vitamin tablets and capsules from the pharmacy in some of my recipes. You can also buy vitamins at natural food stores. Vitamins A and E oils are sold in small bottles and in capsule form. Vitamin C comes in tablet and powdered form.

Water: This is the major component of all living matter and the ingredient most often used in cosmetics. Water is essential for healthy plants and healthy bodies. The best beauty treatment of all is to drink at least eight glasses of water a day! Your skin and hair will glow and you will have more energy. You will also have fewer headaches, which are often a sign of dehydration. Remember always to use the purest filtered water when making cosmetics. If you have questions regarding the purity of the water you are using it is always best to boil it first and then let it cool completely before use in your cosmetic recipes. You do not want to introduce any harmful bacteria or ingredients into your products.

Preserving Your Fresh Ingredients

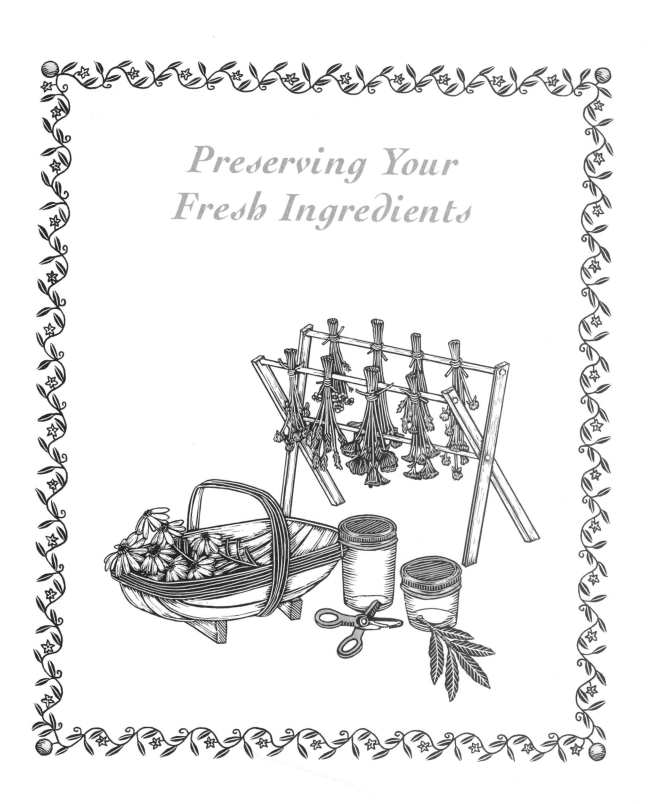

As the growing season comes to a close it is a good idea to take advantage of your garden's bounty or great fresh herb buys. Harvest or buy and preserve these fresh ingredients to use throughout the year in your favorite beauty recipes. Dried ingredients have a more intense flavor and scent than fresh ones. In some recipes, such as those for scented oils, they're also preferred when you do not want additional water introduced into a recipe you are making. Moisture can cause bacteria to grow and spoil the end product. Preserving your ingredients is easy to do and you can choose from several effective, easy methods. The old-fashioned air-drying method is probably the most popular and certainly the simplest to use. Faster ways to dry herbs and flowers involve the use of a food dehydrator or a microwave oven. Freezing is also an option that I have found works well for many fresh leaves and flowers.

The process of drying plants and peels for cosmetic use is similar to that employed for culinary use. It differs from the method used for craft and floral use, as here the appearance of the flowers and herbs is not as important as the quality of the dried plant materials. It is important that the plants you use have been grown without any harmful chemicals, such as insecticides, that could remain on the leaves and flowers. Wash citrus fruits completely to remove any chemical preservatives from their skins. It is also important while drying substances to keep them from becoming dusty. You can prevent this by covering them with cheesecloth or placing them inside paper sacks with slits cut in them to allow air to circulate. You want to avoid any dirt and even small insects ending up in your cosmetic products. Once something is dry it should be promptly put in a clean container. If you hang herbs and flowers for too long, you run the risk that they will become contaminated and lose their usefulness as anything other than a decorative element.

The three main methods of drying are:

1. Air-drying

2. Oven-drying

3. Using a special appliance (microwave or food dehydrator)

The early morning after the dew has dried but before the sun comes out and warms them is the best time to harvest your garden herbs and flowers. The essential oils they contain lose their quality when exposed to heat. Also, you should know that many plants grow from the inside out; the oldest leaves and flowers will be on the outside of the plant. Using sharp scissors, harvest your plants by cutting off the older leaves and flowers. Depending on what you wish to preserve for later, use the leaves of one plant or the flowers and leaves of another. Make sure you label what you collect as some plants look very similar. Be careful to leave at least one-third of the plant so it will continue to grow and produce. Flower petals should be picked after the flower has bloomed but before they drop to the ground. If you purchase fresh herbs and flowers, make sure they have been grown without the use of harmful insecticides because those will remain on the plant. You don't want them anywhere near your skin! Wash your harvested items with cool water and pat dry with a clean towel. Group them by plant type and use the following drying methods to enjoy your harvest throughout the year!

Air-drying is the most popular and easiest. For this, bunch herbs and flowers together and simply hang them upside down to dry. Dark, dry, well-ventilated places work best. If the humidity is especially high where you live, you may want to use a small fan or heater in your drying room. Make bunches small—no more than one inch in diameter—for drying. If you gather too much, mildew may develop inside the bunch. I use rubber bands to bind my bunches together because they contract as the plants dry. Hang these bunches upside down so that all the plant's "energy" flows to the head of the flower or herb and the stems are kept nice and straight. I screwed small cup hooks into the rafters of my garage and hang my plants from them. Wooden clothes-drying racks also work well, and they can be folded up when not in use. Clothes hangers are also good for hanging bunches on, especially if you are using an empty closet for drying. If you're drying many different types of herbs, you may want to tie small paper labels to your bunches. To prevent dust from contaminating your bunches, tie a large paper sack over them. Make sure to cut several slits in the bag to increase air circulation and check the contents often to make sure they are drying.

When your herbs and flowers are crisp and dry, remove the buds and leaves from their stems and place them in clean, dry containers. I have found that glass jars with screw-top lids work best.

For petals and peels you may want to use a drying screen or basket—I have a large, flat, round basket that I use for rose petals. Every time I walk by the basket I give the petals a little stir. In a couple of days they are perfectly dry. You can also make a drying screen from an old picture frame and some clean window screening. Using a staple gun, secure a piece of screen to the underside of the frame. Baskets and screens are good for air-drying because they allow the air to circulate through the plant materials.

Using a conventional oven for drying plant materials is also a good method. It is quicker than air-drying and the problem of dust is greatly reduced. Spread your flowers and herbs on a clean cookie sheet and place the sheet in the center of your oven. Use the lowest possible temperature setting—about 150 degrees Fahrenheit or "Warm." Check every two to three hours. When your herbs or flowers are dry and crisp, let them cool completely and store in clean airtight jars.

Microwave ovens can also be used for drying herbs and flowers. Some manufacturers even list procedures for doing this in the owner's manual. This method works best for small batches of herbs, petals, and peels. What can take two weeks to air-dry can be done in as little as two minutes in the microwave! Every make and model of microwave varies slightly in how it dries, but here is the procedure I use: Place a cup of water in the far corner of your microwave. Lay a paper towel in the bottom of a microwave-safe baking dish. Spread a single layer of herbs or flower petals onto the paper towel, cover with another paper towel, and place the dish in the microwave. Heat the plants for one minute on the lowest setting ("defrost" on my oven). Check and continue heating for thirty-second intervals. Stop if black spots form — that means you're burning them. When your plant materials are dry and crisp, let them cool completely and then package in an airtight container.

Another special appliance that works extremely well for drying herbs, flowers, and peels is a food dehydrator. Many of these come with instructions for drying plant materials, so check your owner's manual before starting. This is a quick, clean method, and because it uses warm air to dry, the plants retain more of their scent and essential oils. Essentially, this is air-drying without the worry of dust. I place whatever I want to dry on the drying racks and use a heat setting of 100 to 130 degrees Fahrenheit. I start my machine in the morning and everything is usually nicely preserved by the end of the day. For safety's sake, remember to turn your dehydrator off if you leave the house.

Freezing is another great method for preserving plant materials. Fresh leaves such as basil, sage, and bay keep well in the freezer. To start the freezing process, first rinse just-picked herbs and flowers and pat dry. Remove leaves and petals from their woody stems. Place them in single layers on baking sheets or foil-covered cardboard and freeze, uncovered, until the items are rigid. This should take about an hour. When you've finished this stage take your materials from the freezer, place them inside freezer containers or resealable plastic bags, and return them to the freezer. The frozen leaves and petals will not stick together. To use, remove only what you need for a recipe. You can easily crumble or chop leaves while they are still frozen. Some herbs, such as rosemary and thyme, may darken slightly when thawed, but this will not affect the outcome of the recipe you are preparing.

After you've used your method of choice for drying herbs and flowers a few things should be kept in mind regarding storage and use. Your dried items are sensitive to heat and strong light. Therefore a cool, dark, dry cupboard is the best place for them. Canning jars and spice bottles with screw lids work best, and you can reuse them. Always label your jars and date them. Dried herbs and flowers can be used in any recipe in place of fresh. The measuring rule of thumb is one-third the amount of dry to fresh; in other words, if your recipe calls for one cup fresh lavender flowers, use one-third cup dried flowers. Drying flowers, seeds, peels, and leaves when particular plants are in season will give you a supply of ingredients to use in recipes all year long.

Gardening Basics

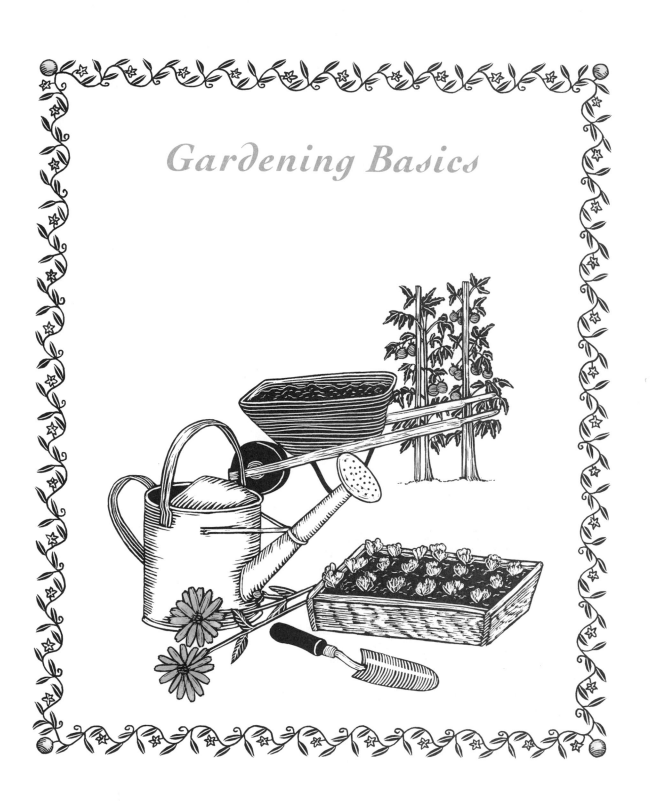

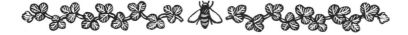

*T*his book is focused on creating natural beauty products from common garden plants. The recipe introductions and garden notes include references to gardening concepts and terms. Also, as any gardener will tell you, we love to share our tips, tricks, and tales, so I have included these as well. You can use this book and create all the recipes and treatments without ever having to grow anything, but if you are inclined to plant a pot, a small vegetable patch, or several acres of fresh flowers and herbs, you should be familiar with a few gardening basics.

Containers and pots: Not all of your plants need to be grown in the ground. Container gardening is very popular, especially for city dwellers and indoor gardeners. A good pot gives you the freedom to create and control your plants. It also makes it possible for each plant to have an ideal growing environment. You can tailor the soil, fertilizer, and even the watering schedule for each individual plant. Containers can also be moved around, which is especially helpful for people living in colder climates. You can simply move the plants indoors during those cold winter months.

Several different types of containers are available in a variety of materials: plastic, terra-cotta, cast stone, and wood. You can use almost any container as long as it can hold water and provides a healthy environment for your plants. This means it should have good drainage, be made out of natural materials so that harmful chemicals will not leach into the soil (some painted containers will do this), and offer enough growing space for your plants. Specialty containers, such as hanging baskets and window boxes, also allow your herbs and flowers to grow in a wide variety of decorative and convenient locations.

Soil: Many people fail to realize how important it is to understand the type of soil they have in their gardens. Soil type and condition are among the most important elements determining how your plants will develop. Knowing what is in the dirt will help you choose what type of plants will grow well and flourish. Garden dirt is a complex biological system made up of air, water, rocks, and organic components. To get a general idea of your soil type, take a sample to your local extension service to have it tested. You can also purchase home test kits and do the analysis yourself. Planting information regarding soil type can easily be found in gardening books, garden catalogs, nursery plant tags, and on the backs of many seed packets. If in doubt it is always a good idea to ask for this information when you are purchasing your seeds and plants.

Compost: Making your own compost has become increasingly popular. Our local disposal company recently offered a deal on garden compost bins and the response was overwhelming. The bins were completely sold out in a matter of hours and the company had thousands to sell! Many communities offer composting workshops and there are several garden books on composting alone. It is popular because it is easy to do, quick, and good for the environment. It also provides an excellent organic soil amendment that will make your garden bloom with health.

All you need to compost is a flat spot in your yard (preferably out of sight) and some organic green and brown ingredients. Brown ingredients are items such as wood chips, small branches, newspapers, dry leaves, sawdust, and straw. Green ingredients are fresh grass clippings, eggshells, vegetable kitchen waste, barnyard manure, and green plant leaves. Never use diseased plants, meat products, or domestic animal droppings in your compost. Layer these materials—green, brown, green, brown . . .—in a pile or special bin. A bin can easily be made with some wire fencing material or wooden slats. Add water to your pile, keeping it moist but not soaking wet. Every couple of weeks give your compost a good turning with a garden fork or hoe to keep air circulating. Depending on your weather and size of your pile, you should have an organic addition for your garden soil in a couple of months.

Finished compost resembles rich, dark soil and does not smell.

Garden tools: As with any craft or activity, the right tools can make all the difference. Gardening is no exception. There are hundreds of items to select from and which ones you decide upon are purely a matter of personal choice. Sometimes my friends and I laugh at the latest garden inventions (especially those sold on late-night infomercials), but then we hear a tale of these tools transforming a neighbor's yard and we all find ourselves longing for these crazy gadgets! There are, of course, some basic tools every home should have: a good garden spade, fork, weeding hoe, rake, pruners, hand trowel, sharp knife, gardening gloves, and watering can. Old tools work just as well and are often sturdier than some of the newer ones, so keep your eyes open for them at garage sales, flea markets, and secondhand shops.

Planting a Container

Once you have decided on your container it is time to plant it. Check with your garden center and purchase a suitable soil mix for your plants. For the best results use a potting mixture designed for containers, rather than soil from your garden. Potting mixtures offer better drainage and a cleaner growing environment. Adequate drainage is important for a thriving container garden. If your container does not have drainage holes, either drill some or add a layer of gravel or pieces of broken pots at the bottom before filling it with soil and planting. A great way to recycle those annoying Styrofoam packing peanuts is in the bottom of your containers. They will keep your pots light and help provide drainage. Mix some organic fertilizer with the soil before you put in your plants. When planting start in the center of your pot and work your way outward, planting your largest plant first. Water your container well to remove any air pockets that may have developed.

You now have a beautiful container garden to grow and enjoy!

Hair Care Products

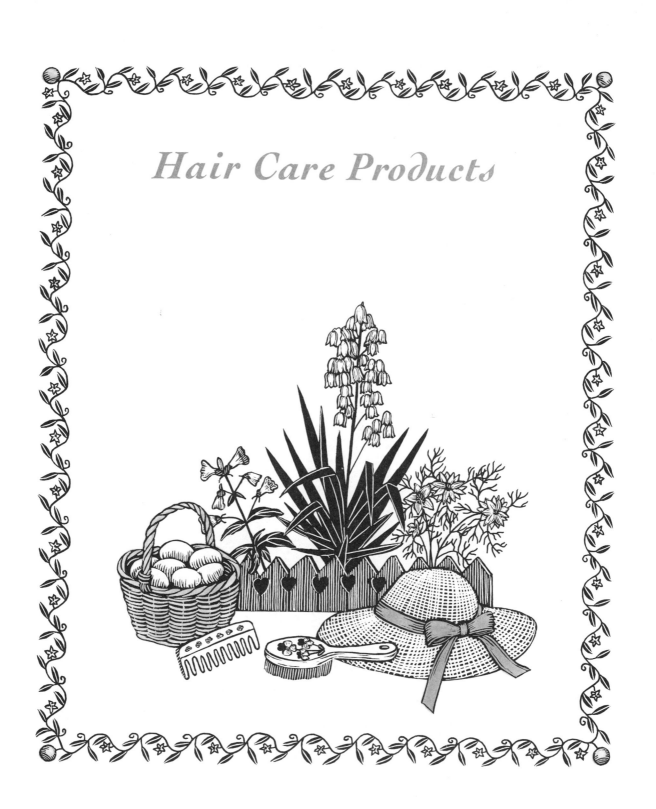

When it comes to our hair it seems we would all like a different texture, color, or style. I hear from readers and friends all the time about their wishes for perfect hair, or hair other than their own. Well, beautiful, healthy, shiny hair can be yours and not some unattainable beauty ideal. The first important step in achieving it is to accept and appreciate the hair you have. It might help to remember that there is always someone out there who wishes he or she had your hair. So whether you have curly, straight, thick, or thin hair, love it, give it proper care, and never wish for another's locks again.

For beautiful, healthy tresses use natural products and practice proper hair and scalp care. To obtain and maintain healthier hair requires long-term effort and attention.

Hair care is really not that different from skin care—the most important things you can do for your hair are to keep it clean and full of moisture. Eating a well-balanced diet, drinking plenty of water, and getting plenty of rest will all be reflected in the glowing condition of your skin and hair. When outdoors, protect your hair with a hat or scarf, for it too can get burned by the sun's rays, which will make it appear dry and lifeless. This is especially important if you dye your hair, as the sun will not only rob it of moisture but also change the color.

Hair care products all perform specific functions that keep your hair looking and feeling its best. This section contains recipes for botanical shampoos, herbal conditioning packs, and rinses that will enable you to say good-bye to bad hair days. There are also recipes for different hair types. If you have very fine, dry hair, try a deep-conditioning hair pack like my Tropical Jungle Conditioner on page 47. It contains fresh bananas and jungle roses. For oily hair, I suggest the recipe for Menthe Hair Rinse on page 54. It is full of fresh mint and is cleansing and refreshing. To cover or darken gray hair a natural rinse of sage, thyme, or rosemary works quite well over time.

Shampoo is intended to clean the scalp first and hair second by loosening dirt and oils. Shampoo is usually a soap-based product with water and conditioning ingredients added, and several recipes for natural shampoo products are included here. There are also recipes for dry shampoos, which come in handy in situations when water may not always be available or convenient. These are practical when camping or at the end of the day for a quick cleaning. (See the recipe for Great Outdoors Dry Shampoo on page 46.)

Conditioning hair packs are similar to facial masks in appearance and are used to restore lost moisture and deep-cleanse your hair. They are rich in natural creams and oils. Massage into your scalp and let the moisturizing ingredients penetrate your hair. Hair packs are especially effective for dry hair and hair that has been damaged by too much sun, blow-dryers, heat rollers, or curling irons. I use a conditioning hair pack weekly, usually applying it in the morning and letting it work its magic as I read our local newspaper, then I jump into the shower. This regular bit of pampering in my weekly routine makes my hair feel incredibly soft and starts the day off right. My favorite recipe is the Clover Honey Conditioner on page 49.

I have also included many natural hair rinses that you can use for highlighting color, cleansing, and conditioning. It seems that everyone I talk to has their own version of a "secret" rinse recipe. Baking soda, apple cider vinegar, and lemon juice all seem to be popular remedies for ridding the hair and scalp of styling product residues. One Canadian reader shared this beauty tip: add a shot of vodka to your shampoo once a week and you will always have shiny, manageable hair. All of my rinse recipes are simple and effective.

Besides getting your hair really clean, a good rinse can also tame flyaway hair or give your hair a bit of color. Chamomile tea makes a wonderful lightening rinse for blondes. Rosemary, sage, and thyme can all be used to bring out highlights in darker shades and cover gray.

Today hair care manufacturers and salons are paying more attention to the scalp by producing products intended for "scalp-only use." This makes total sense, if you think about it. As the source of our hair, our scalp should be well cared for and healthy. Problem conditions, such as dandruff, should be treated; see page 52 for an age-old European cure using fresh garden onions. Everyone can benefit from massaging the scalp, which helps increase circulation and promote hair growth. Try the recipe for Scented Scalp Massage Oil on page 63. New on the market are toners, creams, and lotions intended for the scalp, which, like facial products (and the scalp is really an extension of the face, if you think about it), clean, moisturize, and condition the skin. Try my recipe for Stimulating Scalp Toner on page 40.

Most of us use styling aids such as gels and sprays to help add body to limp hair or to keep our hair in place. But have you tried the natural alternatives that both condition and control? Flaxseed and quince seeds both produce a jellylike substance when soaked in water that can be used as a light, natural styling aid. Jojoba bean oil, used for centuries by Native Americans, can tame unruly manes and give hair an incredible shine. It still beats any modern-day, high-tech commercial product.

Always keep your products in clean jars and bottles. For safety, please do not use glass containers for shampoos and conditioners. These can break if dropped in the shower or bath. Plastic jars and bottles are much safer. I like to use sports-style beverage bottles as they have a handy spout perfect for dispensing shampoos. Store your products in a cool, dark, dry place. Heat and light from a bathroom window may alter the composition of your products. Conditioners that contain fresh ingredients, such as fruit or dairy products, should be stored in the refrigerator.

Love and enjoy your hair!

Stimulating Scalp Toner

¼ cup fresh mint leaves, chopped
¼ cup fresh parsley leaves, chopped
½ cup boiling water
½ cup witch hazel
2 tablespoons vodka

This toner keeps the scalp healthy and clean. It contains fresh mint and parsley, both of which are naturally astringent and refreshing. It gives your head a cooling, tingly sensation that is stimulating after shampooing. You can also use it throughout the day to keep your scalp clean and happy. Fill a small spray bottle with this recipe and spritz the toner onto your hair and scalp for a quick, refreshing pick-me-up.

Place the fresh mint and parsley leaves inside a glass or ceramic container and pour the boiling water over them. Let this mixture cool completely, then remove the leaves by pouring the liquid through a coffee filter or fine strainer. Mix together the parsley and mint water with the witch hazel and vodka. Stir well. Pour the refreshing mixture into a clean bottle with a tight-fitting lid. To use: Pour a small amount onto a clean cotton ball or pad and rub over your scalp. You may also massage it lightly into your scalp with your fingertips.

Garden Note: I left a bag of fresh parsley and mint in my refrigerator and by accident discovered a new and easy way to preserve them. Place your fresh leaves inside a brown paper sack and leave them in the refrigerator. Shake the bag every now and then. In a couple of weeks, the cold air will dry them out while preserving their lovely green color. I think more of the natural oils are retained when you dry herbs this way, as opposed to heat or room-temperature air-drying methods.

Yield: 8 ounces

CHECK YOUR WATER

Did you know that hard water or water with a high mineral content can change your hair color? I have a friend who moved to a country home with its own natural well. Shortly thereafter her beautiful blond hair began to turn orange. After trying different hair products and puzzling over the change, she finally took a sample of her water to the local water agency for testing. It seemed that her well contained a high level of iron, known for its orange hue, and it was the culprit. She installed a water filter on her bathroom faucet and her hair color was restored.

Hard water containing naturally occurring minerals such as iron and copper can stain or discolor your hair. To test your water at home, fill a glass with distilled water and another with water from your tap. Place a teaspoon of dish detergent in each glass. Gently shake or stir the glasses. If the tap water makes fewer suds, then you have hard water and may want to have it checked for mineral content. You can solve the problem of hard water by using a water filter or water softener.

To help prevent mineral buildup and discoloration of your hair you can also use a cleansing rinse, such as baking soda, apple cider vinegar, or lemon juice. Remember, when using acidic rinses such as vinegar or citrus juice, to dilute these ingredients with water. You never want to put them directly on your hair.

Bouncing Bet Shampoo

¼ cup crushed soapwort root and
    leaves
4 cups distilled water

Bouncing Bet" is the nickname given to the herb soapwort. People have used this plant for centuries as a water softener and a gentle wash for skin and hair. In fact, many museums today use soapwort solutions to clean old fabrics, tapestries, and lace because it is so gentle and mild that it will not damage fragile, valuable materials. Soapwort's sweet-scented, pretty pale-pink flower makes a nice addition to any perennial flower garden. Pamper your hair with this ultra-gentle shampoo.

Place the soapwort root and leaves in a medium-size saucepan. Pour the water over them and gently heat the mixture over medium heat for 15 minutes. Strain out all solids and save the soapy liquid. To use: Pour approximately ½ cup over wet hair and massage into the hair and scalp.

Garden Note: Soapwort can easily be grown from seeds. However, once established, these plants can quickly take over your garden. To keep them from self-sowing all over your yard, cut them back after the flowers have faded.

Yield: 32 ounces

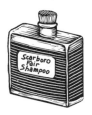

Old-Fashioned Rosewater Shampoo

This is an old-fashioned country recipe of basic household ingredients that have been used by rural women for years to clean and condition their hair. Fresh eggs are a nice moisture-enhancing alternative to soap-based products, which tend to dry out hair. Use cool to warm water when rinsing to avoid ending up with cooked egg in your hair. Make this recipe fresh before each use. You can purchase rosewater or make your own. See Attar of Roses on page 260.

2 tablespoons rosewater
2 tablespoons apple cider vinegar
2 raw eggs

Whisk together all ingredients. To use: Pour half of the mixture onto wet hair and massage into your hair and scalp. Rinse and repeat using the remaining shampoo. Rinse your hair well with cool to warm water. For extra conditioning leave the second application on your hair for 15 minutes before rinsing.

Garden Note: Here are a few tips for cutting fresh roses in the garden: Always cut your flowers before ten o'clock in the morning. Cut above leaflets of five, this will keep your bush healthy and flowering. Make clean-angle cuts with a sharp knife or hand pruner.

Yield: 4 ounces, enough for one shampoo

Alligator Pear Shampoo

½ avocado, mashed
½ cup water
½ teaspoon fresh lemon juice
2 teaspoons avocado oil
½ cup liquid castile soap

Avocado trees originally grew around swamps, which may account for the reason their leathery-skinned fruit was given the nickname "Alligator Pear," a term my grandmother always used. The fruit's flesh is soft and buttery, rich in natural oils and vitamins A and E, making it a well-known beauty ingredient used in rich skin creams, facial masks, massage oils, and shampoos. This recipe is perfect for dry hair types because it contains fresh avocado and avocado oil, which are naturally moisturizing.

Blend together all ingredients. To use: Pour a small amount in your palm to shampoo hair, massaging it into your scalp and through hair ends. Rinse well with warm water. Store any remaining shampoo in the refrigerator and discard after a few weeks.

Yield: 8 ounces

Hopi Bridal Shampoo

½ fresh yucca root or 2 tablespoons
    dried yucca root
2 cups hot water

With their deep green, sword-shaped leaves and tall spikes of scented, tuliplike flowers that bloom after a good rain, yucca plants are found in desert climates. The plant roots produce a soapy mixture when pounded and mixed with water. This astringent soap was used by the Hopi Indians in a ceremony for young brides before their weddings. It cleansed their hair, giving it a healthy all-over shine. You can give your hair this bridal glow every day with the recipe below. If you do not have access to a yucca plant, dried yucca root can be found at most natural food stores.

Place the yucca root in a heavy container and gently pound it to a pulp. Pour the hot water over the mashed root and allow the mixture to sit for several hours. Pour the soapy solution into a clean container; you may strain out the root pulp if you like. To use: Pour over your hair and shampoo as usual. Store this product in a cool, dry location. For a longer shelf life you may want to keep it in the refrigerator.

Garden Note: Yuccas are a wonderful and easy addition to a desert beauty garden. Group them together with aloe vera and jojoba plants. Young yucca plants can also be grown indoors.

Yield: 16 ounces

Scarborough Fair Shampoo

Simon and Garfunkel's 1966 hit song was the inspiration for this recipe. No herb garden is complete without the popular herbal quartet of parsley, sage, rosemary, and thyme. Mixed together with a bit of water and liquid soap, they create a shampoo that makes your hair sing!

Place all the herbs in a glass bowl and pour the boiling water over them. Let the mixture steep for at least 20 minutes. Add the liquid soap and stir well. Pour the mixture into a clean plastic squeeze bottle and let sit overnight to thicken. To use: Pour a small amount into your hand and massage into your hair and scalp. Rinse well with warm and then cool water.

1 tablespoon fresh parsley leaves
1 tablespoon fresh sage leaves
1 tablespoon fresh rosemary leaves
1 tablespoon fresh thyme leaves
½ cup boiling water
½ cup mild liquid soap or shampoo

Garden Note: Urban gardeners can easily plant herbs indoors on a sunny windowsill. Planted individually or mixed together in one container, they will thrive with very little attention.

Yield: 8 ounces

Great Outdoors Dry Shampoo

2 tablespoons orris root powder
    (found in natural food stores,
    often used in making potpourri)
2 tablespoons cornstarch
2 drops rosemary oil (optional)

This dry shampoo removes grease and dirt from your hair when you are unable to wet it. Some people like to use dry shampoos when they are camping and fresh water is hard to find. Dry shampoos are also a helpful alternative for the bedridden or for cleaning wigs and hairpieces. Those of you who have tried them know that using a dry shampoo can be a bit messy. Make sure you are standing on a towel or leaning over a sink when applying one indoors. The rosemary oil I call for here can be made by heating some oil containing a few sprigs of dried rosemary. Let the oil sit for a few days. The longer it sits, the stronger the scent.

Mix together all the ingredients in a glass bowl or resealable plastic bag. To use: Massage a small amount of the dry shampoo powder directly into the scalp and through your hair. You may want to lean over a sink as you apply the powder. Let the shampoo sit for at least 10 minutes to absorb dirt and oils from your scalp and hair. Using a clean, dry, natural bristle brush, brush vigorously, using upward strokes, to remove all of the shampoo. Enjoy the fresh scent of your clean, dry hair!

Yield: 2 ounces

Tropical Jungle Conditioner

A tropical jungle is full of exotic fruits and flowers. This mois-turizing conditioner brings the lushness of the deep rain forest to your shower and is perfect for dry, mistreated hair. It con-tains tropical bananas, which actually grow on large, thirty-foot-high plants, not trees. The dried jungle roses, honey, and macadamia nut oil will hydrate your hair and add extra shine. If you cannot find jungle roses from South America, larger in size than North American ones, any fragrant rose variety will work.

1 cup hot water
½ cup fresh rosebuds or petals
1 medium-size banana, peeled and
    chopped
1 tablespoon honey
1 tablespoon macadamia nut oil
    (if hard to find, use almond oil)

Pour the hot water over your roses and let them sit for a few minutes to wilt and soften. In a blender, combine the banana, honey, and macadamia nut oil. Blend together ingredients on a low setting. Slowly add the rose mixture and continue to blend until you have a smooth cream. To use: Massage the conditioner into your hair and scalp. Cover your head with a plastic cap or piece of plastic wrap. Cover that with a warm towel and allow the conditioner to penetrate for 20–30 min-utes. Rinse your hair well with warm water. Store any remaining conditioner in the refrigerator and discard after a week or two.

Garden Note: Banana plants are big, palmlike perenni-als that seem almost treelike in size. They are easy to care for and fast-growing. A banana plant grown out-doors should be placed in a sunny, wind-sheltered spot and can be grown in a large tub or container. In colder climates, you will want to move the plant indoors for the winter. These giant tropical plants look gorgeous growing next to a swimming pool or fountain.

Yield: 8 ounces, enough for one to two treatments

Rosemary Conditioner

2 tablespoons avocado oil

1 tablespoon castor oil

2 teaspoons strong rosemary tea made from fresh leaves and flowers

2 eggs

This is an enriching treatment for dark hair. It is the perfect hair repair conditioner for damage caused by the sun, water, and wind. Rosemary is superb for putting the luster and life back into your locks. This recipe is full of eggs and natural oils, which are also helpful in conditioning dry or damaged hair.

Whisk all the ingredients together until the mixture is light and airy. Then, using your fingertips, massage the conditioner evenly through the hair and into the scalp. Wrap your hair in a towel and leave on for 20 minutes.

OUTDOOR HAIR CONDITIONING

Give your hair a deep conditioning treatment while you're working in the garden, hiking, or just reading a good book in the sun. Apply a conditioning hair pack, such as the Rosemary Conditioner on this page or the Clover Honey Conditioner on page 49. Comb the conditioner through your hair before heading outdoors. Once you're outside, the sun's warmth will open the hair cuticles, allowing the treatment to penetrate deeply. The hair pack will also help shield your hair from the drying effects of the sun's rays. You may want to add avocado oil to your conditioner recipe, as it has natural UV screening properties.

If you would rather not be seen by fellow hikers or neighbors with conditioner in your hair, cover your head with a cotton bandanna or scarf.

Shampoo and rinse in the normal way. Make a fresh batch each time.

Garden Note: Many people use only the leaves of their rosemary plants, but the flowers are also helpful in making cosmetic products. They have an invigorating scent and contain antibacterial properties, making them ideal for hair conditioners and dandruff treatments.

Yield: 3 ounces, enough for one to two treatments

Clover Honey Conditioner

½ cup pure clover honey (other types may also be used)

Honeybees are nature's best cosmetologists. They produce beeswax and honey, two important beauty ingredients that modern scientists have not been able to duplicate. Pure honey makes an excellent, simple conditioner for dry, mistreated hair. I like to use clover honey because of its lovely scent, but you may use other honey types, such as orange, blackberry, or lavender, in this recipe. This rich conditioner will restore lost moisture, giving your hair added body and shine. If you'd like to lighten your hair, use this recipe regularly. In several months you'll notice its effects. This conditioner may seem a bit sticky at first—but do not worry, it easily rinses out.

Wet your hair with warm water. Massage the honey into your hair, working it through to the ends. Cover your hair with plastic wrap or a plastic shower cap. Wrap a clean bath towel over your hair, like a turban. Leave the conditioner on for at least 20 minutes. Then, shampoo and, if you wish, condition your hair with a light cream rinse, or simply rinse with cool water.

Garden Note: When dealing with garden pests, always try to choose the least toxic control first. For example, aphids on your roses can often be eliminated with a strong spray of water from the garden hose. If you do feel the need to use chemicals, again try to use the most natural ones first and avoid spraying into open flowers. This may harm helpful bees working in your garden. Always make sure you wash your plant materials well before using in cosmetic recipes to remove any residual spray from blossoms and leaves.

Yield: 4 ounces, enough for one hair treatment

Leave-In Irish Potato Rinse

1 cup fresh potato peelings (from about 4 to 5 potatoes)
2 cups cold water
1–2 drops essential oil of rosemary

My father's grandmother came from Ireland where potatoes are a staple of the diet and are grown in almost every garden. Not just for the table, potatoes also had their beauty uses. An old Irish folk recipe for darkening the hair and disguising gray hairs calls for potato peelings. When the fresh peels are boiled the result is a conditioning and darkening hair rinse. Depending on your hair type and color, you may need to use this recipe several times before noticing any color change.

Pour the cold water into a medium-size saucepan. Add the potato peelings and heat the contents over medium heat until the mixture boils. Lower the heat and simmer for 5 minutes. Remove the saucepan from the heat and let the mixture cool. Strain the liquid into a clean container and add the essential oil of rosemary. To use: After shampooing, massage some of the rinse through your wet hair, into your scalp and through your hair ends. Do not rinse. Save any remaining rinse in a clean, airtight container. To extend shelf life, you may refrigerate this rinse. If the rinse begins to smell sour, discard.

Garden Note: Plant nasturtiums near your potatoes to protect them from garden pests. Harmful pests, such as aphids and beetles, will be attracted to the bright flowers, leaving your spuds alone.

Yield: 12 ounces, enough for one to two rinses

Peach Leaf Rinse

Peaches, or Persian apples, as they are also called, are versatile beauty ingredients. Fresh peaches are aromatic and can be mashed into a smooth cream for a luxurious facial mask for dry skin. The oil from the peach kernel, which is inside the peach pit, may be a bit hard to find in some areas but is well worth the effort. It is a light oil similar to sweet almond oil or apricot kernel oil and can be used on all skin types. In this recipe the leaves from the peach tree are used as a rinse to help control fine and unmanageable hair. Rinse the leaves well to remove any orchard sprays.

1 cup fresh peach leaves, rinsed and chopped
2 cups boiling water

Place the peach leaves in a ceramic or glass bowl and pour the boiling water over them. Allow the leaves to steep until cool. Strain off the liquid and pour it into a clean container. To use: After shampooing and conditioning your hair, pour this rinse over your hair. Leave in, and dry and style your hair as you normally do.

Garden Note: Plant catnip near your peach trees to attract beneficial insects to the area and repel harmful aphids.

Yield: 16 ounces, enough for one rinse

European Dandruff Cure

1 medium onion, chopped
½ cup water
1 cup rum

This is a European folk recipe given to me by my German cousin, Elfriede. She swears by it for keeping her scalp healthy, clean, and dandruff-free. Dandruff is one of the most common of all scalp problems and easy to treat. It is characterized by dry, flaky skin on or about the hair roots. The causes of dandruff are many—lack of proper hair care, poor diet, stress, weather changes, and even heredity. This pre-shampoo treatment contains fresh onions, which have the ability to draw impurities from the skin and destroy bacteria. Onions also contain a great deal of sulphur, which is an important mineral for healthy hair. While serious cases of scalp dryness should be treated by a physician, this natural remedy can help cure milder cases with simple handy ingredients.

Mix together the onion and water and gently heat them both until the onion is soft and steamed. You can do this in the microwave. Let the onion cool completely then add the rum. Cover the entire mixture with plastic wrap and let sit overnight. In the morning, strain off all the liquid and discard the onion. To use: Massage a small amount into your scalp before shampooing daily and continue until the scalp is clear and your dandruff is gone.

Garden Note: Onions are easy to grow and are a good companion crop to carrots. Together, they help minimize attacks by both onion flies and carrot rust flies.

Yield: 8 ounces

Sage Tea Rinse

Fresh sage infusions have been used for years to cover silver or gray hair. This treatment is most successful when used over an extended period of time. Sage is probably the best of all plants for darkening and toning the hair. It also has strong antibacterial properties that help keep your scalp clean and healthy. Sage has been used by people for years as a mouthwash, tooth cleanser, and hair growth stimulator.

¼ cup fresh sage leaves
2 cups cold water
2 teaspoons vodka

Gently tear your sage leaves into small pieces and place them in a medium-size saucepan. Pour the cold water over them. Bring the mixture to a boil and remove from the heat source. Let the fresh leaves steep for several hours. Strain off the liquid and stir in the vodka. Pour into a clean bottle or jar. To use: After shampooing your hair, pour this rinse through it and leave in. Do not rinse. Dry and style your hair as usual.

Garden Note: Sage plants like poor but well-drained soil and full sun. They are also drought resistant, making them ideal for hot, dry garden locations.

Yield: 16 ounces

Menthe Hair Rinse

¼ cup fresh mint leaves, gently
    crushed
1 cup sparkling mineral water
1 tablespoon apple cider vinegar

Menthe was a beautiful nymph who caught the eye of the Greek god Pluto. His jealous wife, Proserpine, promptly turned her into an herb and she spent the rest of her life living in the shadows underground, or so the legend goes. This minty rinse will rid your hair of soap residues and restore your natural acid balance, often stripped by modern shampoos, leaving your hair cleaner and healthier than ever. Who knows, you may even attract your own Greek god as Menthe did—just make sure he is single.

Place the fresh mint leaves in a heat-resistant container and pour the mineral water over them. Gently heat this mixture until the water just begins to boil. Cover and let the mixture cool completely. Strain out the mint leaves and discard. Add the apple cider vinegar and stir well. Pour into a clean container. To use: Pour over your hair after shampooing. Let sit for a few minutes and then rinse with the coldest water you can stand.

Garden Note: Mint makes a refreshing iced tea to enjoy on a hot day. Simply pour boiling water over a few fresh leaves, let cool, add ice, and enjoy. This is an excellent way to energize and hydrate your body.

Yield: 8 ounces, enough for one rinse

Eve's Apple Rinse

Ever since Eve offered Adam that first apple in the Garden of Eden, the humble fruit has been known as a symbol of temptation and fascination. But fresh apples also have a less dramatic, but very helpful, use for daily beauty. They make an effective hair rinse that will leave your tresses full of shine and your scalp super clean. Apple juice contains malic acid and amylase, an exfoliating enzyme, both of which help to clean your hair and scalp. The apple cider vinegar also helps to clean the hair and restore your skin's own natural pH level. I hope Eve discovered this beauty recipe before she was asked to leave the garden!

1 large apple, peeled, cut into small pieces
2 tablespoons apple cider vinegar
2 cups water

Mix together all ingredients in a blender or food processor set on "High." Pour the mixture through a strainer into a clean container, discarding all solids. To use: Pour over your hair after shampooing as a final rinse. Massage through your hair and rinse thoroughly with cool water.

Garden Note: Fool Mother Nature and brighten up your winter flower arrangements by forcing flowering tree branches, such as apple, cherry, peach, and quince. Save some branches when you prune your tree and bring them indoors. Place them in vases of water and, after a few weeks, you can enjoy early spring blossoms!

Yield: 16 ounces, enough for one rinse

Country Raspberry Leaf Rinse

1 cup fresh raspberry leaves, washed
2 cups boiling water

Raspberry leaves are naturally cleansing. They have been used by women for years to treat the skin and hair. Fresh leaves make an excellent final rinse for your hair and scalp. They are naturally acidic, which helps restore your hair's natural acid level, which is often stripped away by alkaline shampoos. For a bit of natural color, you may add a few fresh berries to the recipe. If you do not have access to fresh leaves, you can purchase them at a natural food store, or look for herbal teas made from raspberry leaves and use the contents of their bags.

Place the leaves in a ceramic or glass bowl. Pour the boiling water over them and allow the mixture to sit for 15 minutes. Strain and pour into a clean bottle. To use: After shampooing pour through your hair as a final rinse. Dry and style your hair as usual. Save any leftover rinse in the refrigerator.

Garden Note: Ask any raspberry farmers and they will tell you that the secret of growing bushes full of luscious berries is to spread lots of fresh farm manure around them in the spring.

Yield: 16 ounces

Pretty Polly Geranium Rinse

"Pretty Polly" is the nickname given to the variety of scented geraniums that has a delicate almond scent. These plants have attractive light green foliage and large, silvery pink flowers with dark scarlet spots. Used in a hair rinse, the scented leaves lend your hair luster and a lovely natural fragrance. You may also want to try other scented varieties, such as apple, peppermint, or coconut, in this recipe.

1 cup scented geranium leaves, slightly bruised
2 cups boiling water

Place the leaves in a ceramic or glass bowl and pour the boiling water over them. Allow the leaves to steep until cool. Strain the liquid and pour into a clean container. To use: After shampooing and conditioning, pour this rinse over your hair. Leave rinse in; dry and style your hair as you normally would.

Garden Note: Decorate the outside of your pots with paints and stencils, or write the name of each species on your pot's rim with a permanent marker.

Yield: 16 ounces, enough for one rinse

Darkening Hair Rinse

Both rosemary and thyme have been used for centuries to darken the hair and keep it soft and silky. They are also herbs with natural antiseptic properties, which give this rinse the added bonus of keeping your scalp healthy and free of dandruff. After several uses, you will notice the results. Herbal rinses need to build up over time, but the added advantage is that your hair will darken quite subtly and naturally. Your friends may not notice exactly what you did—but they will notice how great you look.

1 tablespoon fresh rosemary leaves
1 tablespoon fresh thyme leaves
2 cups boiling water

Place the herb leaves in a ceramic or glass bowl and pour the boiling water over them. Allow the leaves to steep until cool. Strain the liquid and pour into a clean container. To use: After shampooing and conditioning your hair, pour this rinse over it. Leave the rinse on your hair for at least 20 to 30 minutes (longer if you like). Use a final rinse of two cups cool water, with one tablespoon apple cider vinegar added.

Garden Note: One of my favorite varieties of thyme to grow is lemon thyme. It adds a fresh scent to recipes and has pretty, dark-green glossy leaves.

Yield: 16 ounces, enough for one rinse

Catnip Hair Tonic

2 tablespoons dried catnip or ¼ cup
    fresh leaves
2 cups boiling water

Catnip not only pleases all of your feline friends, it also makes a splendid rinse for your hair. Catnip is part of the mint family and has a pleasant, sweet smell. This scent is what attracts cats, who love to sit and roll around in the plants, much to the disdain of many gardeners. In 1754 a British horticulturist, Philip Miller, wrote this proverb for planting catnip and outsmarting cats: "If you set it, the cats will eat it. If you sow it, the cats don't know it." You can try this age-old garden advice; however, I have found that my cat still seems to find the plants regardless of how they got their start. To keep your young plants safe, sow them in a container placed in a protected "cat-free" spot. In years past, catnip was a valuable crop sold as a curative tea with many medicinal properties. One of its beauty uses is this hair rinse that will help prevent dandruff and give your hair a healthy, glossy shine.

Place the catnip in a large bowl and pour the boiling water over it. Let the mixture cool completely. Strain the liquid. To use: After shampooing your hair pour the rinse water through your hair as a final rinse.

Garden Note: Dry your fresh catnip leaves and stems and use them to stuff little pillows and toys to delight your favorite feline.

Yield: 16 ounces, enough for 1–2 rinses

Calendula Petal Rinse

¼ cup fresh calendula petals or 2 tablespoons dried
2 cups boiling water

Yellow or orange calendula flower petals produce a dye for the hair which was used by European women as early as the sixteenth century. One publication from that time, The New Herbal *(1551), states: "Some women used to make their heyre yellow with the flowers of the calendula plant, not being content with the natural colour which God hath given them." Today calendula petals are used in skin toners, creams, and bath products. They still do make a wonderful highlighting rinse that can be used by both brunettes and blondes.*

Place the calendula petals in a large bowl and pour the boiling water over them. Let the mixture cool completely. Strain the liquid. To use: After shampooing pour the rinse water through your hair.

Garden Note: Make small pots out of newspaper for starting seeds. Roll a few sheets of newspaper around a food can and fold over one end and secure with masking tape. Remove the can. Fill with potting soil and plant your seeds. After your sprouts are several inches tall, plant these containers in your garden. The newspaper will break down and your plants will continue to grow. A beautiful way to recycle!

Yield: 16 ounces, enough for 1–2 rinses

Rhubarb Hair Lightener

3 fresh rhubarb stalks, chopped
1 tablespoon honey
2 cups water

Women have used rhubarb to lighten their hair for years. It is a vegetable, not a fruit, which belongs to the smartweed family and originally came from Mongolia. The stalks grow to be two feet tall, and are a thick and reddish green, each topped by a single, large, umbrella-like leaf. Use only the stalks in this recipe; the leaves should not be used as they are poisonous.

Mix together all the ingredients in a small saucepan and cook over medium-high heat. Bring the mixture to a boil and then reduce heat to a simmer. Simmer for 30 minutes. Allow the mixture to cool completely, then strain. Pour the liquid into a clean container with a tight-fitting lid. To use: Massage about ½ cup of the liquid through clean hair; cover with a warm towel or plastic wrap and leave on for 30 minutes. Rinse your hair well and dry or style as usual. Note: The longer you leave the rhubarb mixture on your hair, the greater the lightening effects will be. You may also need to repeat this treatment weekly for significant color change.

Garden Note: Rhubarb plants last five to eight years and grow best if planted from roots. They produce stalks one year after planting.

Yield: 16 ounces

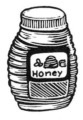

This recipe combines three popular and powerful natural hair highlighting ingredients into one super solution. Chamomile tea brewed fresh from the garden flowers is an old folk recipe for keeping your hair light and blond. In Sweden, pure vodka is the ingredient of choice. I have been told that the purer the vodka, the more dramatic the results. Lemon juice is what I grew up using and is probably the most common of the three. So, whether you choose to use them individually or combined, after a few weeks of applying any number of these ingredients you will have beautiful, naturally highlighted hair, sure to be admired.

Blond Cocktail

1 cup strong chamomile tea
1 tablespoon vodka
1 tablespoon fresh lemon juice

Mix together all the ingredients and stir well. Pour into a clean bottle with a tight-fitting lid. To use: Spray or comb through damp hair before going outside. The sun's rays will highlight and lighten your hair over time.

Garden Note: Chamomile is a great companion plant in the garden. It enhances the growth of cucumbers, loofah sponges, onions, and most herbs. Every garden should contain a patch of these lovely, versatile yellow flowers.

Yield: 8 ounces

GARDEN HATS

Every gardener should have a wide-brimmed hat to protect skin and hair from the elements. The sun can burn and dry out your skin and hair, even in the wintertime. The wind may blow and the rain may fall, but if you have a good hat your head will stay protected. Hats can also become your personal fashion signature for yard and garden days. I have an old raffia hat that I made while living in Australia. This hat has become a part of my gardening wardrobe and I would not even think about going out into the yard without it.

Every now and then it is fun to dress up your hat with a fresh flower or two. This is especially appropriate if you are hosting a garden party. For an easy adornment, pin a fresh flower to your hat's brim with a long florist's pin or hat pin.

For a bit more elaborate decoration, you want to make a complete floral hat band. To do so, start by measuring around your hat's band and add a few inches. Cut a length of raffia or twine to this measurement. Now, beginning at one end, tie flowers and leaves along this string. Sturdy flowers, such as sunflowers, marigolds, zinnias, camellias, and carnations, work well. Green ferns, leaves, and herbs are also a nice addition. This technique is similar to making a garland or wreath. Tie the band around your hat. To keep your band fresh as long as possible, mist it with fresh water daily.

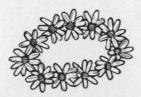

Scented Scalp Massage Oil

A healthy scalp will result in healthier looking hair. A good scalp massage will not thicken your hair or make it grow faster, but it will relax you, ease the pain of a headache, and increase the scalp's circulation and exfoliate dead skin cells and other surface impurities. Australian tea tree oil is a proven antiseptic and helps clean and tone your scalp. I also like to use uplifting and energizing scents in this massage oil, such as peppermint, clove, and lavender, as a mini-aromatherapy treatment.

½ cup light oil (almond, sunflower, or castor oil all work well)
1 teaspoon tea tree oil
2–3 drops essential oil of lavender
1–2 drops essential oil of peppermint
1 drop essential oil of clove

Mix together all ingredients and pour into a clean bottle with a tight-fitting lid. To use: Pour a small amount into your hand and massage into your scalp before shampooing.

Garden Note: Tea trees (*Melaleuca alternifolia*) are an indigenous species of tree to New South Wales, Australia. They are fast-growing, and the oil found within their leaves has powerful antibacterial and antiviral qualities. The tea tree has been used as a medicine plant for thousands of years by Australian Aborigines. Today nearly every Australian household has a small bottle in its medicine cabinet to help heal small cuts, scrapes, and bruises.

Yield: 4 ounces

PRESSED-FLOWER COMBS AND BRUSHES

You can preserve and enjoy your flower petals and leaves by pressing them. Select your favorite blooms then place them between two sheets of waxed paper. To flatten and press your botanicals, place them inside a large, heavy book. In a few weeks they will be dry and ready to use. I like to decorate natural wooden brushes and combs with pressed leaves and flowers. You can do this in a few simple steps.

Glue the pressed flowers and leaves to the back of your hairbrush or comb handle using white craft glue. Let the glue dry and then coat the entire design with decoupage glue or varnish. Repeat, covering your design with at least two coats of finish. Before using make sure the finish is completely dry and hard.

Use your imagination and group your pressed flowers with words, names, and pictures clipped from seed catalogs and magazines. Place them on the flat surfaces of your brushes and combs. You may choose to decorate the entire surface or just the tops and handles of your beauty implements. This is also a great way to save special garden flowers, blossoms from centerpieces, or flowers from bridal bouquets. Each time you style your hair you will be reminded of that special event and the plants and flowers that were a part of it!

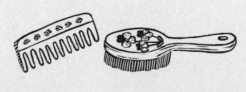

Frizzy hair is no fun. Ask anyone who has thick, curly hair and they will tell you of their desire to tame their unruly manes. I have seen several commercial products on the market that contain high-tech ingredients such as silicone or lightweight polymers that promise to do the trick. These styling aids have their advantages, but cannot compare to good old-fashioned natural ingredients when it comes to conditioning your hair. One of the best is jojoba plant oil. It has been used for centuries to keep hair manageable. Jojoba oil comes from the jojoba plant which grows in the Southwest. It is similar to our bodies' own natural oils and is really more of a wax than oil. Try it on your hair and enjoy the results!

Jojoba Hair Tamer

¼ cup jojoba oil
1 tablespoon light olive oil
1–2 drops essential oil of lavender
  or rosemary

Mix together the two oils and add a drop or two of essential oil for scent if you like. To use: Massage a small amount through your hair. Start at the scalp and work your fingers through the ends of your hair. You may reapply throughout the day, if needed, to keep your hair shiny and smooth.

Garden Note: Jojoba plants (*Simmondsia chinesis*) like full sun and heat and make a handsome clipped hedge for a desert garden. There are male and female plants, so you must have both growing in your yard in order for them to produce the beanlike nuts that provide jojoba oil. Extracting the oil yourself can be done, but it requires some special equipment. It may be more cost-effective simply to purchase your oil.

Yield: 2.5 ounces

Hulda's Setting Gel

2 tablespoons flaxseeds
1 cup distilled water
1 tablespoon rosewater
½ teaspoon glycerine

The Teutons were an ancient Germanic group of people who lived around 100 B.C. One of their legends is the story of Hulda, a beautiful Celtic goddess who taught mortals the art of growing and using plants. One of her favorite herbs was flax. The durable fibers from the stalk of the plant were used in making linen fabric and twine. Linseed oil, made from the small brown seeds of the plant, was used for medicinal purposes. Today we still use flax's many offerings. Flax is an ingredient in modern paper, fabric, paint, linoleum, and cosmetics. In this recipe flaxseeds are used to create a natural hair-setting gel that even Hulda herself would have enjoyed using. Flaxseeds are easy to find in many grocery and natural food stores.

Mix together the flaxseeds and water in a small saucepan and bring to a boil. Remove the pan from the heat and let sit for 15 minutes. Strain the clear, thick liquid into a clean container and discard the flaxseeds. Allow the mixture to cool completely. Stir in the rosewater and glycerine and let the mixture sit overnight to thicken. To use: Apply a small amount, as you would any setting gel. You can use this gel on wet or dry clean hair.

Garden Note: Flax is a very patriotic plant since it produces red, white, or blue flowers in late summer. It is a hardy annual that can grow up to four feet tall. Harvest the shiny brown seeds in the fall.

Yield: 8 ounces

Henna Hair Coloring

Henna is a plant that originally grew in North Africa and Southwest Asia. It has red and white flowers that have a scent similar to roses. The henna you purchase for hair coloring is made from the leaves and stems of this plant. It comes in powdered form, and when mixed together with water creates a paste that can be applied as a hair conditioner and hair dye. Henna is semipermanent hair color, which means it coats the hair shaft and will eventually wear off. An advantage of this is that you will not have noticeable "roots," a phenomenon that can occur with permanent hair dyes. The new color from henna will go through an adjustment period of two to three days. So do not panic if your hair seems brassy or dull right after this treatment—it will soften.

When choosing a color, remember that hair cannot be made lighter with henna. You can make your hair darker by leaving the henna on longer or choosing a darker shade. You can also create new colors by mixing together several different hennas—for example, red and brown henna can be used for auburn hair.

½ cup pure henna powder, using your choice of color (you may need to use more powder if you have long hair)
¼ cup boiling water

Place the henna powder in a ceramic, glass, or plastic container and slowly add the boiling water, stirring until you have a thick paste the consistency of mud. You may need to add a little more water. Do not use metal utensils or containers when mixing henna since some metals, such as aluminum, can react with the plant and cause color changes.

Apply the henna to clean, dry hair. If you are using colored hennas you may want to wear gloves to prevent your hands from staining. Henna powder is available in a colorless or neutral form and is used as a conditioner that will give your hair extra body.

Cover your entire head with the henna and massage well into your hair through to the ends.

Wrap your head in plastic wrap or a plastic shower cap.

Keep your head warm: Sit in the sun, use a blow-dryer and keep it moving, or sit under a warm hair dryer, or wrap your head in a warm, wet towel. Do this for 15 to 45 minutes. The longer you leave the henna in your hair, the darker the color will become.

Rinse your hair thoroughly with warm water until the water runs clear.

Wash your hair using a very mild shampoo and rinse well. You may now dry and style your hair as usual.

Note: Your henna color should last for three to six months, at which point it will have gradually washed out of your hair.

Yield: 2–4 ounces (depending on the length of your hair), or one treatment

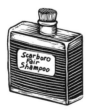

HAIR CARE HERB COLLECTION

Plant a collection of your favorite hair care herbs. Give each plant its own pot and arrange them together outdoors or inside near a sunny window. This makes a simple garden that is easy to handle and move around. When making the recipes in this book you can bring the pot into your kitchen or bath and snip off whatever you need. I would suggest planting:

- **Sage:** This fragrant herb makes a good hair conditioner and darkening hair rinse.

- **Chamomile:** This popular tea herb is known for its hair lightening properties when used over time.

- **Rosemary:** Rosemary hair oil is a popular product because of its conditioning powers. It is also believed to darken your hair color over time.

- **Mint:** If you want to energize your hair, and yourself, use fresh mint in your shampoo, conditioner, and rinse recipes. It is an effective hair beautifier and its scent is a well-known energizer.

- **Lavender:** To deep-cleanse and condition your hair it is hard to find a better choice than lavender. Use the stems, leaves, and flowers in recipes and your hair will shine! Lavender's scent is a well-known body and mind relaxant.

This collection of herb plants would make a wonderful plant gift for a friend, together with a pretty pressed-flower hair brush (see page 64), new garden hat, or some pretty hair accessories.

Facial Care Products
and Treatments

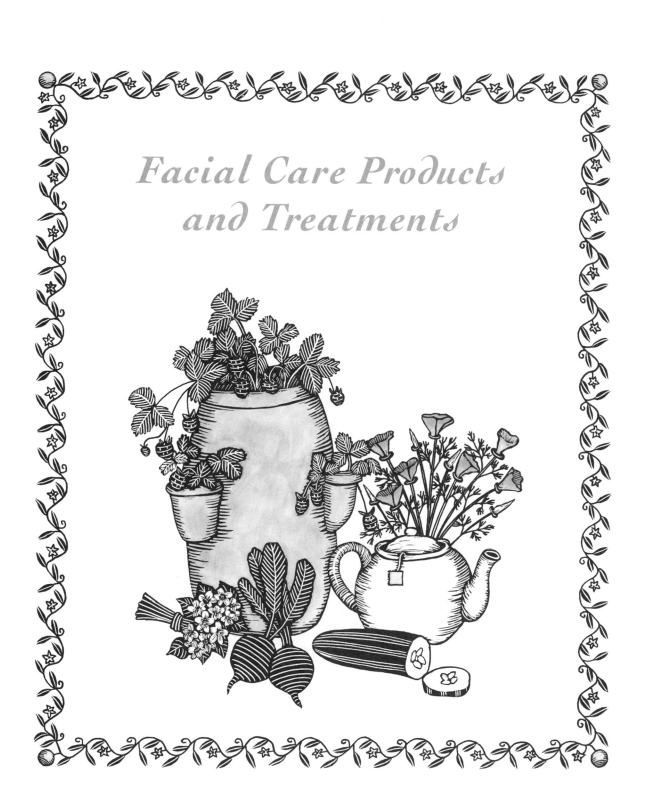

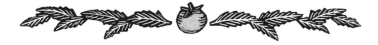

Keeping your complexion healthy and glowing is one of the smartest and easiest things you can do for yourself. Nothing boosts your self-esteem more than clean, healthy skin. It gives you the confidence to do almost anything.

My mother always told me, "Never go to bed with a dirty face." She was right—washing your face in the evening and removing all traces of makeup and surface impurities collected throughout the day is one of the best beauty tips I can pass on.

Several plants you will find in your yard, neighborhood, or market will help cleanse and moisturize your complexion, leaving you looking radiant! Sunflowers, hollyhocks, geraniums, cucumbers, tomatoes, and potatoes are among them. So, grow your own Healthy Complexion Garden as outlined on page 113 and put your best face forward.

Natural cleansers, such as ground oatmeal, sunflower seeds, and aloe vera gel, can help you with this step and are all good alternatives to the classic soap and water wash. You may want to try the Turkish Facial Wash on page 80, which contains fresh beet juice and has been used for centuries by European women.

Cleansing scrubs should also be an important part of your weekly skin care regime. They exfoliate and remove dead skin cells, which improves the texture of your skin and allows it to retain more moisture. I like to use a mild cleansing scrub, such as the Aztec Princess Facial Scrub on page 84. It keeps my skin soft and bright.

Of course, my favorite beauty treatment of all time is the facial mask. It is, after all, what hooked me on home beauty in the first place. When I was twelve, I spread a raw egg on my face and could not believe what it did for my skin. My skin was incredibly soft and smooth. Today, I find there is an added benefit to this simple ritual in the psychological effects it provides. This age-old beauty treatment leaves me relaxed, happy, and feeling beautiful. Pampering yourself for twenty minutes without interruption is quite indulgent, and something we should all do for ourselves for all the benefits it provides.

There are so many fresh facial masks that can be created from plants that I found myself getting carried away. I finally had to limit myself, yet I think the ones in this section are the best! If you try only one, the Alpine Strawberry Mask on page 100 is what I suggest. It will give your complexion an instant boost.

Astringents, toners, and skin fresheners are also important skin care products. They help cleanse the skin of any residue left over from soap or other cleansers. Because many of cleansing products have alkaline properties, it is important to neutralize them and restore your skin's natural acid balance with a rinse or toner. This helps the skin function and combat harmful bacteria that could lead to acne breakouts.

The products that follow cleansing are also extremely refreshing and are great pick-me-ups. Many of my friends use a toner or freshener after exercising if they cannot shower. During the summer months, I like to keep a small spritz bottle of the Chervil Mint Toner, page 93, in my tote bag so I can reach for a mist at any time. It is especially cooling and refreshing on a hot, humid day.

You should follow cleansing and toning with a moisturizing product. Facial creams and lotions are important for complexions because they lock in precious moisture—the key to healthy skin. Dry skin is due to the loss of water, not skin oils. Moisturizing products create a barrier on the skin's surface, locking in water or moisture. Natural plant oils, such as almond, sunflower, or olive oil, are all effective moisturizing products. An excellent recipe to try as you are getting started is the one for California Poppy Lotion on page 110, which is well suited for all skin types.

To help keep your skin protected, remember when you are outdoors to always practice "Safe Sun." A wide-brimmed hat and sunglasses are two of your best beauty tools. Because your face is constantly exposed to the environment, it shows the signs of aging before any other body part. Studies have shown that protecting your skin from overexposure to the sun can greatly reduce the signs of aging. So, to help keep that youthful glow, never go in the garden or outside, even on a cloudy day, without proper protection.

Now it's time to move on to the recipes for all of these facial treatments. I know you'll want to whip up several and have them ready for your daily routine or a little extra pampering. With this in mind, I have included storage suggestions at the end of each recipe. Remember, it is always best to store your products in a cool, dark, dry location. Try to keep your fingers out of the container as much as possible; pour out products, or scoop out creams with a small spoon—this will keep out harmful bacteria and help extend the shelf life of your products. Many of the facial mask recipes are for one treatment. This ensures the freshest product possible each time it is used.

Now, start today by promising yourself to keep your complexion clean and clear naturally. When you feel your best you can accomplish anything!

Four Seasons Facial

I *find a monthly facial is essential for maintaining a healthy and glowing complexion. A facial is a complete cleansing of the skin, and though it may take you up to an hour to complete, it is time well spent. You might even find it an addictive practice. I have outlined a six-step process that involves a facial examination, gentle steaming, massage, facial mask, rinsing, and moisturizing. Your skin should feel as soft as a rose petal when you are finished.*

1. *Examination:* Gently wash your face with a mild cleanser and pat the skin dry. Pull your hair back from your face and examine your skin carefully in the mirror. Is it dry, oily? Take note of blackheads or blemishes and pluck any stray facial hairs with tweezers.

2. *Steam:* Fill your bathroom sink with hot water, then make a tent with a towel and lean forward over the basin. Let the steam envelop your face for 5 to 10 minutes. Gently steam your pores open. You may add a tablespoon or two of your favorite fresh herb leaves or flower petals to the hot water. Note: If you have severe acne, skip steaming. It is not recommended for severely blemished skin; it can aggravate the condition by stimulating blood vessels and activating oil glands.

3. *Massage:* Using your fingertips, gently massage your face in smooth upward strokes. The length of the facial massage depends on your skin type: 12 to 15 minutes for dry skin and as little as 5 minutes for oily skin, to avoid producing more oil.

4. **Mask:** This is the most relaxing part of the facial process. Create a fresh mask based on your skin analysis: For dry skin, a moisturizing mask such as the Moisturizing Honey Avocado Mask on page 104 is a good choice; for oily skin try the Morning Citrus Mask on page 101. Using your fingers or a small pastry brush, spread the mask on your face and neck. Create a thin even layer, avoiding the delicate skin around your eyes. Leave the mask on for 15 to 20 minutes to dry thoroughly.

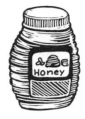

5. **Rinse:** Rinse your face with warm water. Follow with a cool-water rinse for at least one minute, then pat your skin dry.

6. **Moisturize:** Using your favorite facial moisturizer, apply the cream or lotion to your face and neck, and allow it to soak in. Your skin will look radiant, and you will feel relaxed and refreshed!

Galen's Cold Cream

This is a recipe that I have included in all of my books. I do this because it is the basis for all cream recipes and once mastered there is not a cream or lotion you cannot create.

Cold cream, developed by the Greek physician Galen during the second century, has two beauty staples, rosewater and olive oil. It is probably one of the oldest cosmetic recipes still in use today. Ancient Greeks enjoyed the coolness of the cream against their skin, an effect created as the rosewater in the cream evaporated—thus the reason for its name, cold cream. Today women use this heavy cream to remove makeup and keep their skin clean and soft. For an unscented product you may substitute distilled water for the rosewater in this recipe.

¼ cup rosewater or distilled water
⅛ teaspoon borax powder
½ cup olive oil
2 tablespoons grated beeswax

Dissolve the borax in the rosewater in a heat-resistant container and set aside.

Mix together the olive oil and beeswax in another heat-resistant container. Place this container in a pan holding about 1–2 inches of water, making a water bath. Gently heat the oil and wax mixture on the stove or in a microwave oven until the wax is melted; stir well.

Bring the water and borax mixture to the same temperature as the melted wax, hot but not boiling. Again, you may do this in the microwave.

Slowly add the water mixture to the oil mixture, stirring briskly. You may put the two mixtures in the blender and whip, should you prefer. As the mixture cools, continue to stir until well blended and thick.

Pour the cooled cream into a clean container with a lid. It will thicken further as it cools completely. To use: Massage a small amount into your skin and tissue off or rinse off with warm water.

Garden Note: Cold cream can also be used as a rich moisturizer for your hands and feet as you garden. Massage some into your skin before putting on your gloves and boots. This rich cream will protect your hands and feet and keep them from becoming dry and cracked as you work.

Yield: 8 ounces

This cleanser will keep your skin soft and bright. It is a good alternative to soap as it contains two of Mother Nature's favorite herbs for washing sensitive skin: fennel and elderflowers. If neither of these grow in your yard, you may substitute a dried version—just remember to use one-third as much of the dried ingredients because they are more concentrated than fresh ones.

½ cup boiling water
1 teaspoon fresh fennel leaves
1 handful fresh elderflowers
1 tablespoon honey
¼ cup buttermilk

Combine the water, fennel, and elderflowers. Let steep until cool and then strain the mixture. Blend the strained liquid with the honey and buttermilk and store it in the refrigerator. To use: Pour a small amount into the palm of your hand; massage into face and neck then rinse with warm water; pat skin dry.

Garden Note: It is always best to grow plants that will thrive in your environment. If you have a very "wet" area of your yard you may want to plant an elderberry shrub as they grow well in wet soil.

Yield: 6 ounces

Cleopatra's beauty is legendary. The skin care methods she favored have stood up through the thousands of years since her reign. Indeed, many of her ancient beauty secrets are still used today. Aloe vera gel is one. According to numerous ancient writings, Cleopatra attributed her clear complexion to the use of this plant's equally clear gel. Each one of the plant's spiny, lance-shaped leaves holds the soothing substance. The Queen of the Nile used a recipe similar to this one to cleanse, moisturize, and beautify her skin.

2 tablespoons aloe vera gel
¼ cup light olive oil
2 tablespoons rosewater

Blend together all ingredients and pour into a clean container. You may need to stir the mixture before using each time because of its tendency to separate. To use: Massage into your face and neck and rinse well with warm water.

Garden Note: When cutting off aloe vera leaves, always cut from the outside of the plant because the leaves grow from the inside out. Outer leaves, being the most mature, contain the most gel. Harvesting this natural skin soother this way also keeps your plant looking its best.

Yield: 4 ounces

Turkish Facial Wash

⅓ cup fresh beet juice, from approximately 4 small beets
¼ cup rosewater
½ cup distilled water

For centuries, women in Turkey, China, and Egypt have bathed their faces in fresh beet juice to add some color to their cheeks. Inspired by this bit of beauty lore, I mixed up my own facial tonic using fresh beet juice and fragrant rosewater. The result is a gorgeous jewel-colored wash, perfect for adding a bit of glow to pale complexions and can be used to cleanse and tone your complexion. If you do not wish to make fresh beet juice, powdered beet root can be found in many grocery stores, where it is sold as a sweetener. Mixed with water, it is a reliable substitute.

Run the beets through your juicer or food processor and strain. Mix together all the ingredients. Pour into a clean bottle. To use: Pour a small amount onto a clean cotton pad or ball. Gently wipe the facial wash over your face. Do not be alarmed by the bright color—it does wash off. Immediately rinse your face with the coldest water you can stand. Pat your skin dry. Store any remaining wash in the refrigerator. Moisturize your face well afterward with a light natural oil or cream.

Garden Note: The key to successful beet growing is "thinning." When your beet seedlings are 4 inches tall, thin so the remaining plants stand 3–4 inches apart. It may seem hard to do after nurturing the tiny plants, but, trust me, crowded beets do not grow well and will be more prone to pests and disease.

Yield: 8 ounces

POTATO CLEANSER

An easy way to clean the face is to rub it all over with a raw slice of potato. Potatoes contain juice with vitamin C that is mild and soothing, making it an old-fashioned cure for extremely dry skin or eczema. The mild juice thoroughly cleanses and tones your skin; rinse well with cool water after using and pat your skin dry.

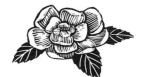

Feverfew Complexion Milk

½ cup fresh feverfew leaves
1 cup whole milk

Feverfew is a two-foot-tall, bushy evergreen perennial that thrives in many soil types. Its yellow and white flowers remind me of small daisies. Feverfew has traditionally been used to relieve migraine headaches when taken as an herbal tea. It also makes a wonderful facial cleanser with the added bonus of nourishing dry skin and helping to remove blemishes.

Place the feverfew and milk in a small saucepan. Gently simmer the mixture for 20 minutes, but do not let it come to a boil. Take the mixture off the stove and allow it to cool completely, then strain. Pour the remaining liquid into a clean container with a stopper or screw-on lid. To use: Massage into your skin and rinse with warm water. Store cleanser in the refrigerator and discard after a few weeks or if the milk spoils.

Garden Note: Feverfew leaves can be picked year-round. However, their scent and essential oil content are strongest just before the plant begins to flower. Keep this in mind when gathering feverfew leaves for your beauty recipes. They may also be dried or frozen for future use.

Yield: 8 ounces

I always know spring is here when I see the sweet violets bloom around my yard. I never planted them; they just appear each year like a gift from Mother Nature for me to enjoy. Cool, moist, and soothing is how my grandmother describes this charming flower. Violets can be added to facial steams, used as a mouth rinse, or added to perfumes. They give this cleansing cream recipe a wonderful, delicate fragrance. You'll find it's a splendid treat for your skin. If you do not have access to fresh violets you may substitute a few drops of violet extract or scented violet oil here.

Mix together the petroleum jelly and oil in a heat-resistant container. Heat until the jelly is melted and the oil warmed. In a separate container, mix together the violets and water. Heat this solution until just boiling. Pour the heated oil mixture into a blender and turn the blender on low. Slowly add the hot violet infusion and continue to blend. You will have a pale lavender colored lotion. Let your cleansing lotion cool completely then pour it into a clean container. To use: Massage into your skin and rinse well with warm water.

Garden Note: Sweet violets will spread each year and are easy to grow. They can be started from runners of already growing plants. Plant them in the early spring, 4–5 inches apart.

Yield: 4 ounces

Violet Cleansing Cream

1 tablespoon petroleum jelly
¼ cup light oil (almond, canola, sunflower)
¼ cup distilled water
1–2 teaspoons fresh violet flowers

Aztec Princess Facial Scrub

½ cup raw sunflower seeds
Distilled water for mixing

Sunflowers are native to Mexico and Peru, where they were once worshipped by the ancient Aztecs who added their floral images to the walls of temples. In the fifteenth century, Aztec sun princesses wore golden crowns of sunflowers. I think they must have stumbled upon the beauty uses of this cheerful plant's seeds as well. This facial treatment can be used to cleanse your skin and leave your face incredibly soft and smooth, due to the rich oil content of the raw seeds. You may also use this recipe for an all-over, full-body treatment.

In a food processor or coffee grinder, process the raw seeds until you have a fine powder that resembles coarse sugar. Pour this powder into a clean container with a tight-fitting lid. To use: Mix one tablespoon of the ground sunflower seeds with a few teaspoons of water to create a smooth paste. You can do this in the palm of your hand or a small ceramic bowl. Massage this mixture into your face and neck and rinse well with warm water first, followed by cool water. Pat your skin dry with a soft towel.

Garden Note: All sunflowers should be planted where they receive a full day of sun. Remember these are very tall flowers, so plant them in the back of your garden or along a fence.

Yield: 4 ounces, enough for eight facial treatments or one full-body treatment

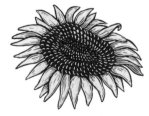

These gentle facial scrubs freshen and stimulate your skin. I like to use the lavender-scented sugar in the morning to brighten my complexion. Use scrubs alone or mixed with a bit of your favorite cleanser. Sugar is gentle enough to use on delicate skin types. It is not as abrasive as it may feel at first since it slowly dissolves as you wash with it. My three favorite scents for scrubs are lavender, vanilla, and basil, but you should feel free to experiment with other flowers and herbs to find your own favorite.

In a clean, dry, glass jar alternate layers of the sugar and dried herbs. If making the vanilla scrub, insert the vanilla bean into the center of the jar of sugar. Cover with a tight-fitting lid or plastic wrap and place in a dry spot for a few weeks. When the sugar is scented to your liking, separate out and save the herbs or vanilla. Don't worry if your sugar has a bit of the herbs or vanilla left in it—I think this actually looks better and adds to this cleanser's homemade charm. Store your sugar scrub in a clean, dry container with a tight-fitting lid. To use: Pour a small amount into the palm of your hand and mix with water or your favorite cleanser. Massage into your face and rinse well with warm water.

Yield: 8 ounces

Scented Sugar Scrubs

¼ cup dried lavender flowers, dried basil leaves, or 1 vanilla bean, split
1 cup granulated sugar

BLEMISHES

Occasional breakouts happen to all of us. Everyone has had the experience of waking up before a big meeting or special event to discover that their skin has erupted almost overnight.

Excitement and stress are two emotions that can trigger your hormones to act up and cause these breakouts. When you are under stress your body secretes extra adrenal hormones, which promote the production of sebum, your skin's own natural moisturizer. This extra oil can block your pores and lead to breakouts. Two ways to avoid these type of breakouts are to relax—a clear head equals clear skin—and keep your skin super clean.

Blemishes fall into two categories: comedones and papules, or blackheads and whiteheads. These types of breakouts occur in your hair follicles, as pores become clogged with sebum and other surface impurities such as dead skin cells and bits of protein. Blackheads are not caused by dirt on the skin, but by excess oil. If this oil isn't removed within eight hours, it hardens into a plug. When air hits the hardened oil, it oxidizes, leaving a black color. If bacteria come into contact with a plugged pore, the result can be inflammation, also known as a whitehead, or the classic pimple. *Never squeeze a pimple; you can cause infection and damage your skin.* Instead, soak a cotton ball in warm salt water and press it on top of the blemish for three minutes to help dissolve the top. Then dab a bit of honey on it and let it sit for another 10 to 15 minutes. The honey helps draw out impurities and has natural germ-killing or antibacterial properties. Rinse with warm water and pat dry.

This fresh cucumber mint toner or splash is perfect for summertime use. I keep it in my refrigerator, which not only extends its shelf life but also makes it cool and refreshing on a hot day. Fresh cucumber juice is also soothing to sunburned skin. The vitamin C I've added to the recipe is a natural preservative. If you cannot find powdered C, simply crush a vitamin tablet with the back of a spoon.

In a blender or food processor blend together all ingredients until liquefied. Strain out all solids and pour remaining liquid into a clean container with a tight-fitting lid. Store in the refrigerator. To use: Splash on clean skin or apply with a clean cotton ball or pad. You may also pour this splasher into a spray bottle and use it to spritz your skin all over.

Garden Note: Cucumbers love to climb. Make sure you plant them next to a fence or trellis so they have something to hang on to as they grow.

Yield: 4 ounces

Summer Splasher

½ *fresh cucumber with peel, chopped (approximately ½ cup)*
½ *cup distilled water*
2 *tablespoons fresh mint leaves, chopped*
⅛ *teaspoon powdered vitamin C*

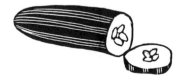

Hollyhock Skin Toner

4 tablespoons fresh hollyhock leaves
1 cup distilled water
1 tablespoon witch hazel

Fresh hollyhock leaves have valuable skin-soothing properties. These old-fashioned flowers were a favorite of Thomas Jefferson, one of our founding fathers. He had several varieties growing in his own garden. Many other flowers and leaves can also be used in much the same way. Lilac and geranium have antiseptic properties; lily-of-the-valley leaves are used for cooling inflammations; honeysuckle promotes healing; lavender leaves have a calming quality as well as a relaxing scent; and dandelion leaves are believed to give your skin added color. You can substitute any of these for the hollyhocks called for in this recipe.

Place the fresh leaves in a small saucepan. Pour water over the leaves and simmer gently for five minutes. Let the mixture stand for 20 minutes, then strain. Stir in the witch hazel. Pour the toner into a clean jar with a tight-fitting lid. To use: Splash on clean skin or apply with a clean cotton ball or pad.

Garden Note: Hollyhocks reseed themselves quite easily. Once these tall flowers are established you can enjoy them in your yard for years without ever planting another seed.

Yield: 8 ounces

Anise is an annual herb that resembles Queen Anne's Lace. It has been cultivated for centuries in Syria and Egypt, where it thrives in the sunny, hot climate. People of the area have used it in perfumes, soaps, facial masks, and mouthwashes for years. Anise seeds, like fennel, have a mild licorice scent and flavor. So, substitute fennel seeds for the anise, if you like. This toner recipe is well suited for all skin types.

1 tablespoon dried anise seeds
1 cup boiling water
¼ cup witch hazel

In a ceramic container, pour the boiling water over the anise seeds and allow them to steep until cool. Strain and discard seeds. Stir in the witch hazel and pour the liquid into a clean bottle with a tight-fitting stopper or lid. To use: Apply to clean skin with a clean cotton ball or spray on skin.

Garden Note: Harvest anise seeds by removing the entire plant head, placing it into a paper sack, and closing it securely. Place the sack upside down in a warm spot, allowing the plant heads to dry completely. This should take a week or two. Once dry, separate out the seeds from the dried flower heads and store them in a dry container.

Yield: 8 ounces

Rose
Geranium
Splash

My favorite of the many scented geraniums is the rose-scented variety. The plant has pretty, pale pink flowers and aromatic green leaves. You can find the oil from these leaves in many health and natural food stores and use it to balance skin oils. The geranium rose oil is antiseptic and has an uplifting scent, which many find makes it an effective and enjoyable skin tonic. I like to use this splash after cleansing my face to tighten pores and reduce any oiliness my skin may have.

1 cup distilled water
1 tablespoon white vinegar
½ teaspoon rose geranium oil

Stir together all ingredients. Pour into a clean container with a tight-fitting lid. You may need to shake this mixture each time before using it. To use: Apply to clean skin using a cotton ball or pad.

Garden Note: Scented geraniums make wonderful indoor plants. Place a few pots inside a sunny window and enjoy the perfume of their leaves. They come in a variety of scents, such as lemon, rose, mint, pine, coconut, orange, apple, and ginger, to name just a few. Use any of these or a combination of them in this recipe.

Yield: 8 ounces

TURN OVER A NEW LEAF

Soak fresh geranium leaves in rosewater, and then put the fresh green leaves onto your face. This should soften your skin and erase wrinkles. Since you will need to lie down so the leaves stay in place, you may want to enjoy a brief beauty nap as well. You will awake feeling renewed and refreshed!

English Tea Astringent

Before my parents left on a recent trip to England, I asked my mother to pick up a few local beauty secrets for me there. She returned with only one—tea! She found that tea is used as a key ingredient in virtually every beauty product, from soaps to shampoos. This isn't really surprising because tea is a powerful antioxidant. With a little research, I found it is an ancient beauty secret that has been used for centuries to cleanse and tone the skin. So, whether your favorite blend is green, orange pekoe, Earl Grey, or jasmine—keep your complexion glowing with a "cuppa" this refreshing astringent.

2 tea bags of your choice
¼ cup boiling water
¼ cup witch hazel
1 teaspoon lemon juice (optional, ideal for oily skin types)

Pour the boiling water over the tea bags and allow them to steep for at least an hour to make a highly concentrated infusion. Combine the cooled tea with the witch hazel and lemon juice. Stir the mixture well and pour into a clean bottle. To use: Apply to clean skin with a clean cotton ball or pad after cleansing.

Garden Note: The tea plant is part of the Camellia family. It is an evergreen shrub with leathery, dull, dark green leaves. It can be grown in warm climates and has small, fragrant white flowers.

Yield: 4 ounces

Cucumber-in-a-Bottle Toner

Small clear-glass or plastic bottle
1 cucumber plant already growing
1–2 cups witch hazel, just enough to
    fill your bottle

I like to think of this recipe as the gardener's version of that age-old craft of the "ship in a bottle." It takes a bit of time to get the cucumber in the bottle, since it has to grow there. But this recipe is fun to share and everyone will want to know how you did it. My daughter took a bottle to school for show-and-tell and inspired several of her classmates to begin their own cucumber projects. Apart from being great fun to make and a real conversation-starter, the toner is gentle and mild and can be used by people of all skin types.

In your garden or a friend's, find a small young cucumber growing on the vine. Slip it inside the neck of your bottle and secure the bottle in place on the vine with a bit of string or twine. Water your plant and watch the cucumber grow inside the bottle (this should take a few weeks). You may need to trim some vine leaves around the bottle neck so that the whole vegetable fits inside the bottle. When you are satisfied with its size, cut the stem of the cucumber, letting it drop to the bottom of the bottle. Fill the bottle with cool water and gently swish to clean off the cucumber and the inside of your container. Pour out the water and fill the bottle with witch hazel. Place a cork or tight-fitting lid on the bottle top. Let the toner sit for one to two weeks before using. To use: Apply to your skin using a clean cotton ball or pad. You may refill your bottle with more witch hazel as you use up the toner. I have noticed the cucumber gets a bit paler the longer it sits in the witch hazel, thus becoming a sort of "beauty" pickle.

Garden Note: Another way to have fun with the cucumber you choose for your toner is to write a message or draw a picture on the fruit's skin with a sharp nail or toothpick. As the cucumber matures your etching will appear for all to see.

Yield: 8 ounces

Chervil Mint Toner

The scent of fresh chervil or "sweet fern," as it is sometimes called, is believed to give one a feeling of well-being. In this recipe it is also used to cleanse the skin, leaving it soft and supple. The lacy foliage of this plant contains vitamin C, carotene, iron, and magnesium. I like to blend it together with fresh mint and rosewater, which are both naturally astringent and help tighten the skin. The result is a refreshing, scented product that helps discourage wrinkles.

¼ cup fresh chervil leaves
¼ cup fresh mint leaves
1 cup boiling water
¼ cup rosewater

Place the chervil and mint leaves in a glass or ceramic bowl. Pour the boiling water over the leaves and let the mixture sit until completely cooled. Strain the mixture and discard all solids. Mix this solution together with the rosewater and pour into a clean bottle with a tight-fitting lid or stopper. To use: Apply to your skin with a clean cotton ball or pad.

Garden Note: Since I suggest using fresh leaves for the best toner results you may want to grow your own chervil. Put the plant in light shade for the most fragrant foliage. It can also be grown indoors quite easily.

Yield: 8 ounces

Oregon Elderflower Water

Elderberry trees grow wild along the Oregon country road to my parents' home. During the summer months I pick their creamy white flowers to enjoy their delicate, muscat aroma. These blossoms later turn into tiny, sweet black berries. Elderflowers have a refining effect on the skin and are useful in many facial skin care products, such as toners, eye creams, and moisturizers. This simple recipe is one of my favorites.

½ cup fresh elderflowers
½ cup vodka
¼ cup witch hazel

Mix together all the ingredients in a glass jar and let sit for one to two weeks. Strain out the elderflowers and pour the astringent into a clean container with a tight-fitting lid. To use: Apply to your skin with a clean cotton ball or pad.

Garden Note: Elderflowers can be gathered in June and July and air-dried for year-round use. Gather only the flower blossoms and discard the leaves and twigs. If you are not lucky enough to have an elderflower tree in your yard, you may find them in the wild growing along country roadways. If you gather them on property other than your own, make sure they have not been sprayed with any harmful insecticides—and that you have permission to pick them.

Yield: 6 ounces

Hop Flower Astringent

2 tablespoons fresh or 1 tablespoon
   dried hop flowers
¼ *cup boiling water*
2 *tablespoons vodka*

Some women put fresh beer directly on their skin to keep it clean and clear. I prefer this homemade beauty brew made from fresh hop flowers. Hops are grown mainly for the brewing industry; they are added to beer to flavor, clarify, and preserve it. The plant takes its name from the Anglo-Saxon word hoppan, *meaning to climb, which this plant can surely do. These vines are easy to grow, but be warned they can grow to over 20 feet! Hops have large green leaves and cream-colored flowers that have a delicate beerlike scent. You may also purchase dried hops in many natural food stores or beer-making supply shops.*

Place the hop flowers in a ceramic or glass dish. Pour the boiling water over them and let them steep until completely cool. Strain out the solids and add the vodka to the hop liquid. Stir well and pour into a clean container. To use: Apply to just-washed skin with a clean cotton ball.

Garden Note: If you have a problem with slugs and snails destroying the plants in your garden, invite them over for a beer. Pour a little beer into a small container, and place it in your garden so that the edge is just even with the soil line. Slugs and snails will crawl in for a drink and then drown.

Yield: 3 ounces

In Germany, chamomile daisies grow in almost every garden. There is a phrase for this well-loved herb in that country— alles zutraut, *meaning "capable of anything." In fact, around the world chamomile is often referred to as the "physician's plant" because it has so many health applications. This aromatic evergreen has strong anti-inflammatory and disinfecting qualities, and is also soothing to wind-chapped or sunburned skin. This recipe will soothe and calm your complexion and can be made as easily as a cup of tea.*

In a ceramic container, pour the boiling water over the chamomile and allow it to steep for at least three hours. Strain out the flowers and pour the resulting liquid into a clean container with a tight-fitting lid. To use: Apply to clean skin with a clean cotton pad, or spray on skin. Let dry.

Garden Note: Chamomile is a creeping herb, with the stems rooting themselves as they spread. It makes a fragrant lawn substitute and smells glorious when mowed.

Yield: 8 ounces

German Chamomile Tea Soother

½ cup fresh chamomile flowers or 2 chamomile tea bags (made from 100 percent chamomile flowers)
1 cup boiling water

Potato Mask

¼ cup fresh potato juice (juice of
one medium peeled potato)
¼ cup white China clay (kaolin
clay) or fuller's earth

You say "pa-ta-toe," I say "po-tay-toe"—however you pro-
nounce it, let's just call it a wonderful skin soother! This light
creamy mask is well suited for oily skin types. The natural clay
(see page 107 for a description of the clays used in this recipe)
absorbs excess oil and surface impurities from the skin and
adds the benefits of potatoes, which are well-known skin beauti-
fiers. Potato juice can easily be made in the blender or a juice
machine. Simply liquefy chopped potatoes and strain out all
solids. You will want to make this mask fresh each time, as it
does not store well. It will turn a reddish brown when left sitting
out uncovered.

Stir together the potato juice and clay with a fork until
well blended. To use: Spread the mask over clean skin
using your fingertips or a small brush. Let sit for 15 to
20 minutes, or until dry. Rinse well with warm water
and pat your skin dry.

Garden Note: Potatoes are ripe when the tops of the
plants become withered and yellow. Do not worry that
your plants are dying; they are just signaling they are
ready for harvest.

Yield: 2 ounces, enough for one facial mask

Alexander the Great Banana Mask

Alexander the Great was king of the Macedonians and one of the most famous generals in history. During their conquest of India in 327 B.C., he and his troops discovered a wonderful, nourishing new food—the banana. This rich, creamy fruit was a welcome addition to the warriors' diet. Today the banana is the number one fruit enjoyed around the world. Used in many creams and hair products, it is also an important beauty ingredient. In this recipe it is used as a splendid facial mask, perfect for dry skin. For normal skin types you may want to omit the sunflower oil. It may simply be too rich for oily skin types, so if your skin falls into this category I would not recommend using this mask recipe.

½ mashed ripe banana
1 teaspoon sunflower oil (or any light oil)

Stir the mashed banana in a small bowl with a fork until smooth and creamy. Add the oil and mix well. To use: Spread the mask on clean skin using your fingertips or a clean brush. Leave on for 10–15 minutes. Rinse well with warm water and pat your skin dry. Discard any remaining mask, as it will not keep.

Garden Note: Don't throw that peel in the trash! Add your banana peels to the compost bin, as they provide potassium, or spread them under rosebushes to ward off aphids.

Yield: Approximately 2 ounces, enough for one facial mask

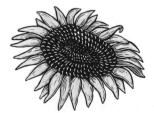

Roman Fennel Mask

¼ cup boiling water
1 tablespoon fresh fennel leaves, finely chopped
1 tablespoon pure honey
2 tablespoons plain yogurt

Fennel was much valued by the Romans. Gladiators ate it for good health before battle. Ladies often ate it to alleviate hunger and prevent obesity. Every part of the plant, from the seeds to the root, had a use. Ancient Romans also knew the benefits this herb provided for the skin and added fresh fennel to their baths and complexion waters. In this recipe the aged herb is combined with plain yogurt and honey to create a deep-cleansing facial mask that will leave your skin incredibly soft.

Place the fresh fennel in a glass or ceramic bowl. Pour the boiling water over it and let the mixture cool completely. When cool, strain off the liquid. Mix together the fennel water, yogurt, and honey. To use: With a small pastry or art brush, apply the mixture to clean skin. Let sit for 15–20 minutes. Rinse your skin well with warm water followed by cool and pat your skin dry. Store any remaining mask in the refrigerator.

Garden Note: Do not plant fennel next to dill or coriander as they will cross pollinate, thereby reducing the fennel seed production.

Yield: 2 ounces

Ophelia's Rosemary Mask

½ cup distilled water
1 tablespoon fresh rosemary leaves
2 tablespoons oatmeal

In Shakespeare's Hamlet, *Ophelia is the beautiful sister of Laertes who is drawn into a plot to expose Hamlet's madness. In the play, she mentions the herb rosemary many times, the most famous of these lines being: "There's rosemary, that's for remembrance; pray, love, remember." Ophelia was a victim of rottenness in Denmark, but her practice of aromatherapy was right on target. Fragrant rosemary is a well-known memory enhancer. It is also a wonderful skin toner. So use this mask to condition both your mind and your complexion. It is perfect for all skin types.*

Mix all ingredients together in a blender and process until smooth. Pour the mixture into a heat-resistant container and heat gently until just boiling. For this step I use the microwave on high for 2 minutes. Allow the mixture to cool and thicken before using. If your mask comes out too thick to spread easily, add more water and stir well. To use: Spread the mixture on clean skin and let sit for 20 minutes. Relax. Rinse the mask from your skin using warm water; pat your skin dry. Store any remaining mask in the refrigerator.

Garden Note: I keep a small pot of rosemary indoors on my desk. Whenever I need to gather my thoughts I snip off a few leaves and focus on its memory-enhancing fragrance. Its unique smell, and mind-prompting properties, have helped me time and time again. Try it for yourself!

Yield: 4 ounces

Pineapple Sage Mask

I have a pineapple sage plant in my yard that I love—not for its fresh tropical scent, or downy green leaves, or even its easy care—although it has all of those lovely things. What beats all of these attributes is the wonderful, bright scarlet, flame-like flower that instantly brightens an otherwise dull spot in my yard every autumn. Sage is a well-known hair rinse, but it also makes a wonderful facial mask, perfect for all skin types. Any type of sage will work in this recipe, but I love to use pineapple sage for its delicious scent!

½ cup boiling water
1 tablespoon fresh pineapple sage
   leaves (or other sage varieties)
3 tablespoons oatmeal
2 tablespoons pure honey
1 egg white

Pour water over the sage leaves and allow to cool completely. Strain, and add the sage liquid to the oatmeal, honey, and egg white. Mix well until smooth and creamy. Spread the mixture on clean skin and let sit for

15–20 minutes. Rinse well with warm water and pat your skin dry.

Garden Note: Pineapple sage is a perennial herb that can grow to 3 feet in height. It likes well-drained soil and full sun. Cut back the stems in the fall after flowering and it should last for several years. You can start new plants from stem cuttings to share with friends.

Yield: 2 ounces, enough for one facial mask

Alpine Strawberry Mask

½ cup fresh strawberries, mashed
1 tablespoon plain yogurt or sour cream

In Europe, small red berries grow wild in the alpine meadows where they thrive on the limestone soil. These sweet berries came to be known as strawberries. A member of the rose family, they are rich in salicylic acid, a common ingredient in many commercial products for troubled skin. This fresh strawberry mask deep-cleans your skin and removes any surface impurities. If you have blemishes, this is a good mask to try. It leaves the skin smooth and tight. It is also a soothing treatment for sunburned skin.

Mix together both ingredients to make a smooth paste. Spread over your face and neck and let sit for 20 minutes. Rinse with warm water, followed by cool water. Pat your skin dry. Refrigerate any leftover mask and use or discard after one week.

Garden Note: Strawberry plants can be grown in hanging baskets. With their cheerful white blossoms and juicy red berries they are a welcome addition to any porch or patio area.

Yield: 4 ounces

Acne Rosacea Treatment

I was given this recipe by one of my readers, who swears by its anti-inflammatory powers. Acne rosacea is severe facial flushing, a common skin problem that usually affects fair-skinned individuals. Turmeric and coriander, or Chinese parsley, have strong anti-inflammatory properties. It is important to note that if you have been diagnosed with this skin condition, it is best to check with your physician before starting any new type of treatment. So, talk with your doctor before using this mask.

2 teaspoons dried turmeric powder
4 teaspoons dried coriander powder
1–2 tablespoons fresh milk

Mix together the powdered herbs with enough milk to form a smooth paste. Bring the paste to a boil on the stove or in the microwave. Once it has boiled, remove from the stove and cool completely. To use: Twice a day, or when flushing occurs, apply the mixture to your face and neck and leave on for 10 minutes. Rinse well with warm (not hot) water, followed by cool water, and pat your skin dry. Store any leftover product in the refrigerator and discard if the milk spoils.

Yield: 1 ounce

Morning Citrus Mask

As an orange lover, I was lucky growing up in Southern California, and had two grandfathers and a father who grew oranges—fresh-squeezed juice was always on our breakfast table. This refreshing morning facial mask uses fresh citrus and is the perfect way to start your day. I like to spread the mixture on my face and read the morning paper—it is more refreshing than a cup of coffee! Oranges contain citric acid, making this mask well suited for troubled or blotchy skin. If you have sensitive skin you may want to do a patch test (see page 9); you should not leave this mask on your face for more than five minutes.

1 egg white
juice of ½ orange, approximately ¼ cup
1 teaspoon fresh lemon juice

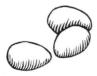

Beat the egg white until white and foamy using a small whisk or fork. Add the orange juice and lemon juice and mix well. Spread the mixture onto clean skin and leave on for 5–10 minutes. Rinse with cool water and pat your skin dry. Discard any remaining mask; it does not keep well.

Garden Note: Any fruit tree makes a lovely shade tree for your yard. Growing them near your house enables you to enjoy the fragrant blossoms they provide and allows you to see when the fruit is ripe and ready to pick.

Yield: 2 ounces, enough for one mask

Fresh Carrot Mask

¼ cup fresh carrot juice, made from approximately 2 large carrots
¼ cup white kaolin clay (China clay)

The orange-colored roots of the carrot plant are rich in vitamin A, often referred to as the "beauty" vitamin because of its importance in maintaining healthy skin and hair. Fresh carrot juice has strong antiseptic qualities, making it an excellent ingredient for a facial treatment for blemished skin. You may purchase fresh carrot juice, or make your own using a high-speed blender, food processor, or juice machine. For extremely dry skin, add one teaspoon of light oil to this recipe.

Mix together the carrot juice and clay until smooth. For a thicker mask you may add more clay. To use: Spread the mixture on clean skin using your fingertips or a small brush. Let sit for 20 minutes, rinse well with warm water followed by cool, and pat the skin dry. Store any remaining mask in the refrigerator for up to one week.

Garden Note: Carrot seeds take some time to germinate and it is sometimes easy to forget where you have planted them. A simple solution is to plant radishes along with your carrots. They grow very quickly, marking your planted row. You can harvest your radishes when the carrots begin to sprout.

Yield: 2 ounces, enough for one to two masks

Love Apple Mask

2 tablespoons yellow cornmeal
1 tablespoon French green clay
1 tablespoon fresh tomato juice
1 tablespoon distilled water

Tomatoes were given the nickname "love apples" during the seventeenth century. The story is that Spanish conquistadors, returning home from exploring Peru, brought with them a new useful plant. The people of Peru called it "tomata." It soon became known in Europe by its Italian name, "pomodoro," which the French interpreted as "pomme d'amour," or love apple. Today the tomato is one of the most popular garden plants, grown all around the world. Fresh tomato pulp is awfully tasty, but did you know it can be used as a refreshing and cleansing facial mask? That's right! The pulp is mildly acidic and it helps rid your skin of excess oil that can cause breakouts. For sensitive skin you may want to use the less acidic yellow tomatoes. The cornmeal in this recipe will help clear your pores of any surface impurities.

In a glass or ceramic container mix together all ingredients and stir well until you have a smooth paste. To use: Spread the mixture onto clean skin, gently massaging with your fingertips. This will help exfoliate any dead skin cells and other surface impurities. Leave the mask on your skin for 10–15 minutes, then rinse with warm water. Discard any remaining mask.

Garden Note: Tomatoes are some of the easiest garden vegetables to grow. Urban gardeners should look for varieties that can be cultivated in containers and hanging baskets.

Yield: 2 ounces, enough for one facial mask

Moisturizing Honey Avocado Mask

½ *fresh avocado, approximately*
⅓ cup
1 teaspoon pure honey

This is my favorite mask for hydrating extra-dry skin. It combines two super ingredients that make excellent facial masks by themselves — honey and avocado. Honey is a natural humectant that keeps your skin full of moisture. Avocados are full of natural oils and protein, both beneficial to your complexion. Whenever my skin looks extremely dry and I can actually see dry patches in the mirror, I use this recipe. After just one application, my skin is visibly softer and smoother.

Mix together both ingredients until smooth and creamy. To use: Massage the mixture into your face and neck. Let sit for 20 minutes then rinse well with warm water. For extra-dry skin you may leave the mask on overnight: After massaging mixture into your skin, tissue off any excess. I would also suggest using an old pillowcase, or cover yours with a light cotton towel to avoid ruining good bed linens. Store any leftover mask in the refrigerator. It may darken a bit but this will not affect its use.

Garden Note: Avocado plants grown from the pits of store-bought fruit make excellent houseplants. However, the mature, pit-started trees bear fruit a bit different in shape, size, and quality. If you are interested in planting an avocado tree in your yard, I would suggest starting with a young tree from a local nursery.

Yield: 3½ ounces

Your Own Avocado Tree

During the late '70s the California Avocado Advisory Board had an advertising campaign with the slogan: "Inside every avocado there's a free tree." I took this ad to heart and would never let an avocado pit fall into the garbage. As a result, at one time I may have had twenty trees growing in my bedroom! As my virtual grove of trees illustrates, the avocado planting process is simple. Next time you have an avocado, save the seed and let the tree sprout out!

Here is how:

1. Wash the seed in tepid water.

2. Drive three toothpicks into it and suspend (broad end down) over a jar, covering only ½ inch of seed with tepid water.

3. Place in a warm spot out of direct sunlight. Give the seed about 2 to 6 weeks to root.

4. When the stem reaches 7 inches, cut it in half so it branches out. Once roots are thick and the stem has leafed out, carefully plant in potting soil, leaving the seed half exposed. Use a large pot with good drainage.

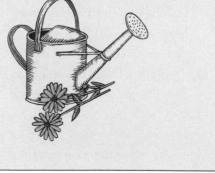

Single-Ingredient Masks from the Garden

There are dozens of fresh masks that can easily be made using one type of garden-fresh produce. Here are a few of my favorites:

Cucumber: Fresh chopped cucumbers (you can leave the peel on) make a gentle, toning mask for all skin types. This is an especially soothing and cooling summer treatment. Cucumber juice is also a good cure for sunburned skin. Pat fresh cucumber juice onto your burned skin and leave on for 15–20 minutes, then rinse well with cool water.

Parsley: Finely chopped, parsley is soothing to blotchy or troubled complexions. To deep-cleanse and freshen normal-to-dry skin add some parsley to a few tablespoons of sour cream, or for oily skin to a well-beaten egg white. Spread the mixture onto your face and leave on for 15–20 minutes. Rinse well with warm water.

Corn: Because of its high fat content, corn milk (made from grating fresh corn over a bowl) is soothing to extremely dry skin. Pat on the skin and leave on for at least 20 minutes. Then, rinse well with cool water.

Rose hips: Rose hips are the fruit of the rose and are usually harvested in the fall. They are small, orange-red fruits, about the size of a small cherry, and are found just below the rose flower. Dried and powdered rose hips are available at many natural food stores. They are rich in vitamin C and can help calm and clear the skin. To make a facial mask, crush the rose hips and mix them together with some rosewater or distilled water until you have a smooth paste. Spread the mixture on your face and neck and leave on for 10 minutes. Rinse off with cool water and pat your skin dry.

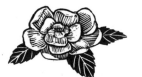

Garden Note: Rose hips are picked in the late fall, just before the frost destroys them. All roses have "hips," but only certain species of the rose have a fruit suitable for eating. *Rosa rugosa* is the most common fruit-bearing variety in the United States.

Natural Clay Masks

Clay or mud masks are some of the oldest natural beauty treatments still employed today. People have used the earth for centuries to deep-cleanse the skin. Usually a wet mud is made by mixing naturally occurring clay with water, which is then applied to the face or the entire body. As this mud dries it draws out oils, surface impurities, and dead skin cells, leaving the skin soft and smooth. Clay masks can also be used on the hair to deep-cleanse and condition it. It is important to note that you never want to use earth directly from your yard these days, because it can contain harmful bacteria. It is best to purchase sterilized clay from your natural food store or pharmacy. Here is a sampling of some of the more common clays you will find:

2 tablespoons natural clay
1–2 tablespoons distilled water

Fuller's earth: A fine gray clay that comes from algae found in seabeds and river bottoms.

Kaolin clay: Sometimes called "China clay," this is a fine white powder originally obtained from Kaolin Hill in China.

French green clay: A fine, pale-green clay that comes from southern France.

Bentonite: A volcanic white clay found in the midwestern United States and Canada.

Rhassoul mud: A red clay from the Atlas Mountains in North Africa.

Mix your clay mask fresh each time using equal parts clay and water. Stir well until you have a smooth paste. To use: Spread the mixture on clean skin and leave on for 15–20 minutes, until dry. Rinse well with warm water followed by cool water and pat your skin dry.

Yield: 1 ounce, enough for one facial mask

British Eyebright

2 tablespoons dried eyebright leaves
1½ cups boiling water

This herb has been used since the Middle Ages to refresh, soothe, and brighten the eyes. During Queen Elizabeth's time it was also used as a memory tonic and as an ingredient for making ale. Eyebright is a dainty little plant with small, deeply cut leaves and tiny, pale lilac-colored flowers. It grows wild in meadows and pastures across the British Isles. It can easily be found dried in many natural food stores. Use this recipe to soothe tired eyes with a cool compress. After a brief nap, your eyes will sparkle.

Place the dried herb in a ceramic or glass dish. Pour the boiling water over it and let sit for 15 minutes. Strain and pour the liquid into a clean container. Refrigerate until cold. To use: Dip sterile cotton pads in the solution and place over your closed eyes. Lie down and rest for 15–30 minutes. Store any leftover solution in the refrigerator.

Yield: 12 ounces

Refreshing Eye Gel

This cool, clear gel is perfect for soothing and moisturizing tired eyes. Use it in the morning under makeup or at the end of the day for a quick pick-me-up. It contains fresh cucumber juice, aloe vera gel, and witch hazel, which are all naturally astringent and cooling.

1 tablespoon aloe vera gel
1 teaspoon fresh cucumber juice
¼ teaspoon cornstarch
1 tablespoon witch hazel

Mix together the aloe vera, cucumber juice, and cornstarch. Heat until just boiling. This usually takes one minute on high power in the microwave. Remove from your heat source and stir in the witch hazel. Stir well and allow the mixture to cool completely. You should have a clear, jelly-like cream. Spoon into a small clean jar. To use: Dab a small amount under your eyes and be careful not to rub or pull the delicate skin under your eyes.

Garden Note: When growing cucumbers, pick them often. This will keep your plants high-producing and healthy.

Yield: 1 ounce

CUCUMBER CLASSIC FOR PUFFY EYES

This is an easy age-old beauty tip shared by women around the world for refreshing the eyes and reducing under-eye puffiness. It works because fresh cucumbers are naturally cooling and astringent.

Go out into the garden or open up the refrigerator and grab a fresh cucumber. Slice off two thin slices. Lie down and place the cool cuttings over each eye. Relax. After 10–15 minutes under-eye puffiness will be reduced and you will feel restored.

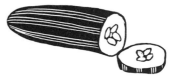

California Poppy Lotion

⅓–½ cup fresh poppy flower petals
1 cup boiling water
⅛ teaspoon vitamin E oil

The state flower of California is one of my favorite perennial wildflowers. The golden-orange flowers appear to be made of tissue paper because they are so fine in texture. This simple poppy lotion is surprisingly effective. It may seem a bit watery in appearance, but it will make your skin feel like velvet. I like to use it on my face after washing in the morning. It also makes a nice, light body lotion.

Remove the flower petals from the flower heads and rinse gently. Place in a glass or ceramic bowl. Pour the boiling water over the petals and stir in the vitamin E oil. Let the mixture cool and steep for several hours or even overnight. Strain and pour into a clean container with a tight-fitting lid. To use: Splash the lotion on your face and body and gently massage into your skin. Do not rinse.

Garden Note: Poppies are among the easiest flowers to grow from seeds and as such are a perfect choice for beginning gardeners. Simply scatter the small black seeds around your yard and delight in the bright flowers they produce.

Yield: 8 ounces

Hungarian Tomato Lotion

In Hungary, women rub fresh tomato halves over their faces to clean and tone their skin. After hearing this European beauty secret, I was inspired to create this recipe from one of my favorite garden fruits. Tomato juice is rich in lycopene, a powerful antioxidant much like vitamins C and E. It helps to refresh and tone your skin. It also improves your circulation, which as you know is very important for glowing skin.

⅛ teaspoon borax powder
¼ cup distilled water
1 tablespoon fresh tomato juice
   (you may also used canned)
½ cup light olive oil
1 tablespoon grated beeswax
⅛ teaspoon vitamin E oil

Mix together the borax, tomato juice, and water, and set aside. Place the olive oil, beeswax, and vitamin E oil in a heat-resistant container and warm until the beeswax is melted. Stir the oil mixture. Warm the tomato juice solution until it is the same temperature as

REFRESHING RAINWATER

"If you walk barefoot through the morning dew, you will become beautiful." This is a bit of American folklore that could be true, since going barefoot will certainly put a smile on your face. For years women have used dew or rainwater to wash. Country women have always preferred rainwater from the barrel to well water, as it is softer on the skin and hair. Collect your own rainwater for washing or to make your favorite recipes. Simply place a clean bucket or container outside in the rain. You may want to boil the water you gather to make sure it is sterile. Allow it to cool completely before using. Another way to enjoy a rainy day is by walking face up for a healthy and stimulating rainwater facial massage.

the oil mixture. Place the oil mixture in a blender and mix. In a slow steady stream add the tomato juice solution and blend. Pour the lotion into a clean container and allow to cool completely. To use: Massage a small amount of this rich lotion into your skin.

Garden Note: To increase your tomato harvest always pinch off the sucker shoots that appear in the "V" of the plant branches. These will never produce fruit, yet they take valuable energy and nutrients from your plants.

Yield: 4 ounces

Floral Facial Steam

2 cups water
¼ cup fresh rose petals
¼ cup fresh camellia petals
¼ cup fresh lavender flowers

A flower petal facial steam is a good way to remove city grime and air pollution from your pores. The heat and humidity gently open your pores, allowing impurities to escape. Fresh flower petals create a fragrant facial steam that will keep your skin soft. I like to use a combination of rose, lavender, and camellia petals, but lime flowers and elderflowers also work well. You may also substitute flowers with your favorite fragrant herb, such as mint, basil, sage, or rosemary, all of which are a bit more astringent.

Please note: Steaming is not recommended for badly blemished skin. It can aggravate the condition by stimulating blood vessels and activating oil glands. If you have a continuing skin problem you should check with a physician or dermatologist before trying.

Boil water in a covered, medium-size saucepan. After bringing the water to a boil, remove from heat, add the flower petals, and stir. Let the mixture sit for 5 minutes. Lean over the pot—at least 12 inches from the surface—and drape a towel over your head to form a tent.

Close your eyes and let the steam rise over your face for 5 minutes. Rinse with cool water and pat dry.

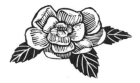

Garden Note: Pick your flowers in the early morning — just after the dew has dried — for the most fragrant blooms.

Yield: 16 ounces, enough for one facial steam treatment

HEALTHY COMPLEXION GARDEN

Plant a small corner of your yard with flowering plants, herbs, and vegetables as your own private complexion garden. Growing your own plants is not only enjoyable but you will be assured of fresh, pesticide-free ingredients for all of your beauty recipes. Working outdoors in the fresh air tending your plants is also good for your skin. I suggest starting with the following plants:

Cucumber: Easy to grow from seeds, these love to climb, so plant them near a fence or give them their own trellis to grow on. Fresh garden cucumbers are a beauty must; they are mild and refreshing for all skin types.

Tomato: Young plants can be found at many nursery centers in the spring. For unusual varieties, you may want to start from seed. Tomatoes are best used on oily complexions in masks and facial scrubs. Some less acidic yellow varieties can be used by individuals with normal skin.

Fennel: This is easy to grow and can quickly take over a small section of your garden. Fennel is mild enough for all skin types when used in cleansers and facial toner recipes.

(continued)

Hollyhock: These tall flowers are wonderful in facial toner recipes. They come in a variety of colors—even black for those urban New York gardeners. They are easy to grow and will come back year after year. Birds love to plant these flowers for you all around the yard.

Chamomile: Chamomile is an all-around beauty herb used in creams, lotions, toners, and many hair products. You cannot beat chamomile for its gentle nature and effectiveness at calming a complexion breakout.

Sunflower: These garden giants make you feel good just looking up at their sunny faces. Their seeds are excellent skin scrubbers, and their petals can be used in making cleansing facial toners and astringents.

All these plants are easy to grow and thrive in most climates. You may start your garden from seeds or purchase small plants at your local garden shop.

Mouth Care Products

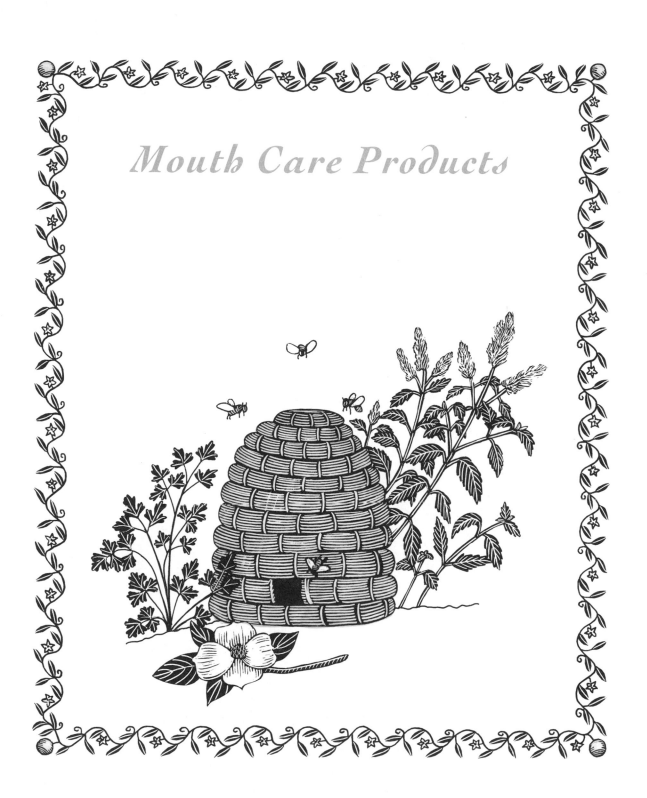

The mouth is at the center of some pretty important activities such as eating, drinking, breathing, and kissing. Not to mention my all-time favorite—talking! It is also a feature of beauty. How many times have you heard, "He has such a wonderful smile," or "When she smiles it lights up a room!" People have understood the importance of the mouth for centuries. The ancient Egyptians painted their lips. Native Americans used simple toothbrushes made of twigs. The use of natural breath fresheners and mouth rinses is universal.

A healthy smile is one of your best beauty assets. I am a firm believer in proper mouth, teeth, and lip care. These are parts of our bodies we cannot easily cover up. It is important that our teeth and gums remain clean and healthy, our lips soft and full of moisture, and our breath fresh and sweet smelling.

In this section you will find recipes for tooth powders, mouth rinses, and lip balms and glosses. All of these products are useful for beautiful, healthy mouths. They will create a mouth that will get noticed—for all the right reasons!

Our teeth are about the most durable part of our body. They have to be. We use them constantly. We only get two sets of teeth in our life, so proper dental care is critical. Brushing and flossing are two of the most important things you can do for your teeth. This helps rid your teeth of harmful bacteria or plaque that can break down the tooth enamel and cause decay. Use a good tooth cleanser, such as the recipe for Fresh Peppermint Toothpaste on page 128, and brush for at least two full minutes. While you are brushing your teeth, don't forget to brush your gums to keep them healthy. Equally important to brushing is flossing—even the best toothbrush cannot remove the plaque that gets under the gums and between the teeth. Regular dental checkups and professional teeth cleanings are a must. This is especially critical if you smoke, or drink coffee or tea. All three can stain your teeth.

Nothing is more embarrassing than halitosis or bad breath. My husband, who has perfect dental habits, always points out when my breath is less than lovely. Even though his habit is sometimes annoying, it is also quite helpful. It is difficult to smell your own bad breath because your nose adapts to any odor you're exposed to over time. Because of this fact, it is best to ask someone about the state of your breath if you are unsure.

Cleaning the mouth often and keeping it moist and fresh will help reduce any offensive odors. Dry conditions are a contributor to bad breath. This is where the term "morning breath" comes from. After a night of sleeping our mouths are drier because saliva production slows down. Talking on the phone for extended periods of time, exercising, skipping meals, and the use of certain medications also dry out the mouth. A dry mouth can be avoided by drinking plenty of water or water-based beverages such as herbal teas that boost your mouth's saliva production. Using a fresh mouth rinse such as Lavender Mouthwash on page 126 will also help. It is important to note that chronic bad breath may be a symptom of another health problem. If it persists, please check with your physician.

The best insurance for a sweet-smelling, healthy mouth is brushing your teeth, gums, and tongue. Brushing the tongue can help your breath stay fresher longer. Brushing your teeth and tongue kills twice as many bacteria as just brushing the teeth. This is probably the reason for all those high-tech tongue scrapers on the market. (I have found a soup spoon works just as well. Simply insert the spoon upside down and press the edge down into the tongue. Rub it across the surface several times, then rinse your mouth well with plenty of water.)

Another part of our mouths that needs special care is our lips, one of the most sensitive areas of the body. They are vulnerable to weather conditions and excessive moisture. Proper lip care is similar to good skin care. Protection is very important. The use of a good lip balm or gloss such as Red Clover Lip Gel on page 121 helps to form a layer on top of your lips, locking in moisture and preventing them from drying and chapping. It is also a good idea to use a sun block on your lips when outdoors, as lips, too, can burn. Try the recipe for Aloe Vera Lip Gloss on page 123. Some people have the habit of licking their lips. This should be avoided, as it actually dries out the lips, causing them to chap and crack. If your lips do happen to crack, you can easily exfoliate them. Gently cover your dry lips with a layer of light vegetable oil, then scrub them gently with a warm, wet washcloth or soft toothbrush. Protect them with more oil or your favorite lip balm recipe.

Lipsticks and lip stains have been used throughout history as cosmetic products. The earliest known lip color dates back to 3500 B.C. It was made by the Mesopotamians from a base of white lead. It was in Paris in 1910 that lipstick as we know it today was first introduced. Now it is the most commonly used and most frequently purchased cosmetic product in the world. My own mother never leaves the house without first applying a bit of color to her lips.

Lip glosses and balms are easy to make. Their production mainly involves melting together a few ingredients and letting the whole mixture cool. At home you can achieve some natural tints with garden ingredients such as beet juice, rose petals, and fresh berries. It is hard to duplicate darker, commercial lipstick brands without purchasing expensive pigments (they can be ordered from suppliers). Many of my friends grate a bit of their favorite commercial lipsticks into their recipes for a bit of added color. I prefer more natural shades and love the transparency of glosses. They add a subtle color to the lips and give them lots of shine.

The care and storage of these products is simple. Tooth powders should be stored in clean, airtight containers and kept dry until used. Discard any powder after it has been mixed with water. It is always best to mix up a fresh amount with each use. Mouth rinse products that do not contain alcohol and are made with fresh ingredients will keep longer if refrigerated. Lip stains, glosses, and balms all have long shelf lives but will last longer if they are scooped out of the container with a clean cotton swab, lip brush, or small spoon. If you do use your fingertips as an applicator, make sure they are clean. Always store your products in cool, dark, dry locations. Excess heat may cause your lip products to melt. If this happens, stir well and place in a cool spot, or even put inside your refrigerator.

Keep smiling!

Red Clover Lip Gel

This is an old folk remedy for dry, chapped lips. Red clover is commonly found in country gardens and fields. It has three green leaflets and a red-purple flower. The flowers yield a sweet honeylike substance that has anti-inflammatory and skin-soothing properties. Dried flowers are easily found at any natural food store due to their popularity in making herbal teas.

½ tablespoon dried red clover
    flowers, or 1 tablespoon fresh
¼ cup water
¼ teaspoon clover honey
⅛ teaspoon vitamin E oil
⅛ teaspoon cornstarch

Combine the clover flowers, water, and honey, and bring the mixture to a boil using either the microwave or stove. Boil for 2 minutes then remove from the heat source and strain the liquid. Stir in the vitamin E oil and cornstarch, mixing well. Heat this mixture until it forms a clear gel (1–2 minutes). Cool this gel completely, stirring occasionally. Spoon into a clean container. To use: Spread on your lips.

Garden Note: Many gardeners think of red clover as a weed. It seems to pop up in moist, grassy areas. Its cousin, white clover, is often grown for hay.

Yield: ½ ounce

Pineapple Sage Lip Cream

Fresh pineapple sage flowers, with their tropical scent and mild fruit flavor, are a wonderful addition to this rich lip cream. You may also substitute other fresh herb flowers, such as lavender, thyme, or cinnamon basil, in this recipe. I like to use this lip cream under or over colored lipsticks for extra shine and protection.

½ tablespoon grated beeswax
1 tablespoon sesame oil
½ teaspoon jojoba oil
1 teaspoon dried pineapple sage
    flowers, or 2 teaspoons fresh

In a heat-resistant container place the wax, oils, and sage flowers. Heat the mixture until all the wax is melted. Pour through a strainer into a small, clean jar or lip balm container and discard any solids. Lip balm containers can be purchased at pharmacies or ordered from cosmetics supply shops. Let the mixture cool completely until solid. To use: Rub on your lips with a clean finger or lip brush.

Garden Note: Cut the bottoms off plastic milk jugs and place them over small plants to protect them from frost.

Yield: ¾ ounce

Apiarian Lip Balm

2 tablespoons grated beeswax
1 teaspoon sunflower oil
1 teaspoon apricot kernel oil
⅛ teaspoon vitamin E oil

The word apiarian *means pertaining to bees. It comes from* apiary, *which is where bees and beehives are kept. Gardeners have long appreciated the bee for its importance in pollination. Many old-fashioned gardens have a beehive or apiary placed in a corner to encourage the busy insect to take up residence. This lip balm uses a valuable product from the beehive—wax. It can be used alone or under lipstick to keep your lips soft and protected.*

In a double boiler or microwave, gently melt the beeswax and oils together and stir well. Pour into a clean lip balm container or small plastic box and allow to cool completely. To use: Apply to your lips.

Garden Note: Welcome bees into your garden by planting bee-attracting herbs. They love rosemary, thyme, catnip, chamomile, flax, sage, fennel, calendula, marjoram, parsley, lemon balm, and bee balm. These busy insects will happily pollinate your plants. A nearby beehive can increase your garden yield by 50 percent!

Yield: 1½ ounces

Strawberry Jam Gloss

Everyone appreciates homemade jams and jellies. Each summer my daughters and I like to cook up batches so we have enough to give throughout the year as hostess gifts. We also like to create this sweet-tasting lip gloss. It is made with fresh berries and will give your lips a delicate pink color.

1 tablespoon almond oil
1–2 fresh strawberries (approximately 1 teaspoon)
½ teaspoon honey
¼ teaspoon vitamin E oil

Mix together all the ingredients and place them in a microwave-safe or heat-resistant container. Heat in the microwave or a double boiler until the mixture just begins to boil (1–2 minutes in the microwave). Stir well and gently mash the berries into the mixture. Let sit for 5 minutes. Strain the mixture through a fine sieve to remove all pieces of strawberry. Stir and allow to cool completely. When cool, spoon into a clean container. To use: Simply spread a small amount on your lips.

Garden Note: Strawberries are one crop with which it pays to be patient. Each year they will produce more and more. The first year pinch off all the blossoms as they appear. This stimulates the plants to spread and multiply.

Yield: ½ ounce

Aloe Vera Lip Gloss

This light gloss will protect your lips and give them extra shine and moisture. Aloe vera gel is soothing to your skin because of its high water content. If you have an aloe plant growing in your home, use its gel in this recipe. To gather the gel, cut off one of the larger leaves near the plant's base (aloe plants grow from the center out), split the leaf lengthwise, and scrape out the clear jelly into a small dish. You can also buy bottled aloe vera gel at many health and nutrition stores.

1 teaspoon fresh aloe vera gel (or packaged)
½ teaspoon coconut oil
⅛ teaspoon vitamin E oil

Mix together the aloe vera gel and oils, and stir well. Pour into a clean lip gloss container or small jar. To use: Apply a small amount to your lips using a clean fingertip or lip brush.

Garden Note: Aloe plants are not only contributors of a soothing gel, they also have striking flowers that bloom in the winter months. These flowers are usually orange in color but also come in red and pink varieties.

Yield: ½ ounce

Fresh Spearmint Lip Gloss

1 teaspoon fresh spearmint leaves
2 teaspoons light oil
1 teaspoon grated beeswax

I like to use fresh spearmint in this recipe but other varieties of mint would also work well. You may want to try orange, pineapple, cinnamon, or chocolate.

Place the leaves in a glass or ceramic container. With the back of a spoon, gently bruise the leaves. Pour the oil over the leaves and cover with plastic wrap. Let this mixture sit for several days. For a stronger scented oil, you may remove and replace the leaves each day. Remove all mint leaves from your oil. Mix the mint oil with the beeswax. Gently heat the mixture until the beeswax melts, stirring well. Pour the melted gloss into a clean container and allow it to cool completely. To use: Apply to your lips.

Garden Note: Mint is one of my favorite garden plants because of its exhilarating scent. If you do not want your mint to take over your yard—they are prolific spreaders—keep your plants in containers.

Yield: ½ ounce

Everyone has at one time or another sampled the fresh parsley garnish on their plate while dining in a restaurant. It is placed on your plate to add a bit of color and is one of the most effective herbal mouth fresheners around. Now, you may or may not enjoy parsley's fresh, very green taste—not everyone does. So here is a list of several other fresh leaves, flowers, and berries for you to sample. Many nutritionists agree that eating an herbal mouth freshener after a meal is good for you, since the stomach is where many mouth odors originate. Here is a list of some tasty fresheners to try:

Fennel leaves—mild licorice flavor

Peppermint leaves—fresh and, of course, minty

Sage leaves—savory flavor helps digest fatty foods

Parsley leaves—fresh green flavor

Pineapple sage flowers—fruity tropical flavor

Basil leaves—warm spicy flavor

Juniper berries—bittersweet flavor also helps digestion

Thyme leaves—antiseptic taste, used in commercial mouthwashes (Thymol). I like using lemon thyme.

Rose petals—delicate floral flavor

Lavender leaves and flowers—fresh, clean flavor

Garden Note: At your next dinner party place an edible herbal garnish on your guests' plates. Choose one that can be enjoyed at the end of the meal and will also freshen everyone's breath.

Lavender Mouthwash

1 tablespoon vodka
2 tablespoons rosewater
1 cup boiling water
1 tablespoon fresh lavender leaves

Lavender leaves freshen the breath and clean and disinfect the gums. This is a mild, almost tasteless mouth rinse that has an airy floral fragrance. You can also use this as a skin freshener or after-bath splash. This is especially helpful when you are traveling and you want to avoid carrying several different products. Both lavender and rosewater are naturally antiseptic.

Place the lavender leaves in a glass or ceramic dish and pour the boiling water over them. Let this mixture steep for several hours then strain, and discard the leaves. Add the vodka and rosewater to the scented liquid. Stir well and pour into a clean bottle. To use: Pour a small amount into a clean glass and rinse your mouth after brushing your teeth and gums.

Yield: 8 ounces

Raspberry Chocolate Mint Mouthwash

Eating fresh berries such as strawberries and raspberries will whiten and clean your teeth. This is due to the berries' high content of natural fruit acids. This rose-colored mouthwash has a fresh taste and is a great way to sweeten your breath. It smells good enough to eat, and you can! (It makes a refreshing morning drink.) It is also alcohol-free, which many people prefer as it is gentler on your teeth and gums.

Place all the ingredients in a blender and process on "High" until well mixed. Pour the liquid through a strainer and discard all solids (bits of mint leaves and raspberry seeds). Pour the liquid into a clean container. To use: Swish one to two tablespoons in your mouth. Note: Discard if mouthwash begins to smell or taste sour. To extend shelf life, store in the refrigerator.

Garden Note: Fresh berries can easily be preserved by freezing them. I use the following method so that the fresh berries do not become one solid mass: Spread your berries on a cookie sheet covered with wax paper. Place this sheet in your freezer. When the berries are frozen solid, pour them into resealable containers or plastic bags.

Yield: 16 ounces

1–2 tablespoons fresh chocolate mint leaves (about 5 small sprigs)
5 fresh raspberries (you may use frozen)
2 cups mineral water
1 500-mg vitamin C tablet, crushed

Fresh Peppermint Toothpaste

1 tablespoon fresh peppermint
leaves (three small sprigs)
¼ cup cold water
½ teaspoon sunflower oil
½ teaspoon cornstarch

The cool, clean taste of peppermint is a classic toothpaste flavor. This pale-colored gel is made using fresh mint leaves and will help clean both your teeth and gums. It is nonabrasive, making it a good choice for people with sensitive teeth and gums.

Gently tear the fresh mint leaves and place them along with cold water in a small saucepan or microwave-safe container. Bring the mixture to a boil, remove from heat, and allow to cool for 15–20 minutes. Mix together the cornstarch and oil, and stir until smooth. Strain the mint leaf solution, and discard the leaves. Mix together the mint water and cornstarch mixture. Bring this mix to a boil and then cool, stirring occasionally. Spoon the cooled mixture into a clean container. To use: Spread a small amount on a clean toothbrush and brush as usual.

Garden Note: Most mint will grow almost anywhere except in hot, direct sun. Mint does best in light, rich soil that is moist and in the shade. Keep mint flowers pinched back to encourage bushy growth. I do this by making small arrangements for my home with these tiny minty flowers.

Yield: 2 ounces

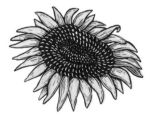

Dogwood Toothbrush

This recipe is a bit of botanical beauty trivia. It is good to know if you are outdoors and need to clean your teeth. Flowering dogwoods, or Cornus florida, *are gorgeous, showy trees that in the spring are covered with creamy white or pink blossoms. (These pastel petals are actually leaf bracts, rather than flowers on the tree branches.) You can create a simple, natural toothbrush from a flowering dogwood tree. It is important to use freshly cut twigs as they are more soft and pliable for cleaning the teeth and gums. I like to dip my dogwood brush in some baking soda, which acts as a simple toothpaste.*

1 4-inch freshly cut twig from a
   flowering dogwood tree
Water
Baking soda (optional)

With a sharp knife peel about one inch of bark from one end of your twig. Chew on the end until it is soft and frayed, creating a "brush." Gently rub the brush over your teeth and gums. You can dip the twig in water and then in some baking soda. Store your twig in a cup of fresh water and discard after a few uses. It is best to use a fresh stick each time.

Yield: 1 toothbrush, one to two uses

KEEP SMILING CONTAINER

Plant a small container with parsley, mint, and sage. This mouth-freshening combination of herbs can be used in beauty recipes or as a centerpiece for your next outdoor dinner party. Simply eat a few leaves to freshen your breath and cleanse your mouth. You may also want to plant one for your bathroom. Keep it next to your sink and enjoy a few leaves after brushing your teeth for sweet, fresh breath.

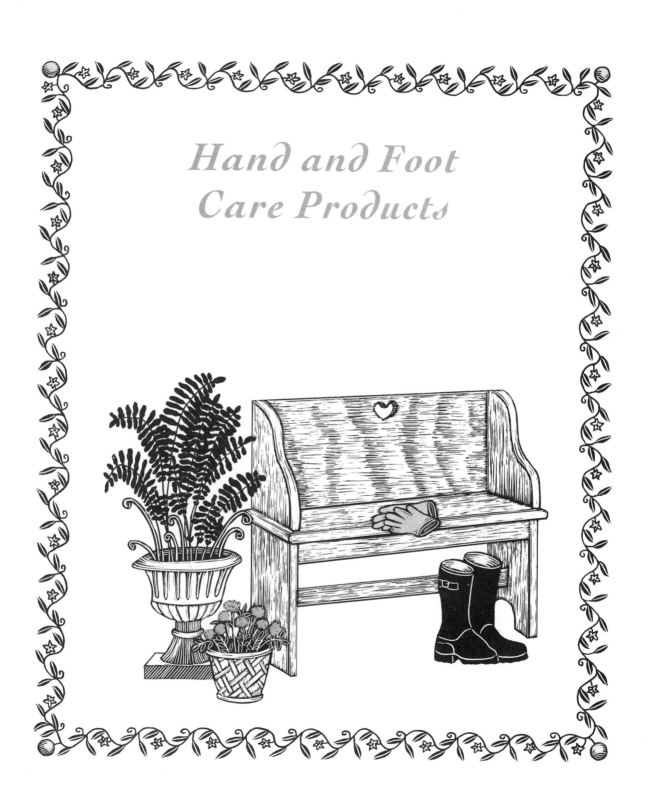

Hand and Foot Care Products

When we are working in the yard or garden, our most important tools are certainly our hands and feet. It seems when something needs to be pulled, picked, hauled, or planted we depend on them to get the job done. These hardworking body parts deserve proper care and protection. They are helpful, strong, and dependable—it is up to you to keep them looking and feeling their best! This section contains the products and treatments to do just that.

Manicures and pedicures are two wonderful beauty treatments to do by yourself at home. Be even more indulgent by performing them in your garden surrounded by your green plants and fragrant flowers. In this section I have included step-by-step instructions for both of these pampering treatments. I have also included recipes for hand creams, nail strengtheners, cuticle creams, foot creams, and foot baths. All of these will keep your hands and feet looking well cared for.

Healthy and strong nails are really easy to have. With just a bit of common sense care and a little pampering they will look truly lovely. Eating a proper diet is essential for healthy nails. A diet with too little protein can make your nails dry and dull. In addition, your nails are extremely porous, so it is important to keep them full of moisture. My grandmother makes a conscious effort to apply a rich cream to her hands and nails after each time she washes them. This helps form a protective coating that locks the moisture into her hands and nails. I try to practice this same beauty routine. Cuticle creams, like the recipe on page 140, help increase your circulation and promote nail growth. Remember, never use your nails as a tool for scraping or prying something. It is always best to go get a screwdriver or knife rather than ruin your nails.

I've also included a section on garden gloves. Wearing protective gloves will help keep your hands clean and soft. Many people say you can tell real gardeners by the condition of their hands. I disagree—real gardeners use gloves and do not get "green thumbs." Proper glove selection will keep your hands as beautiful as the flowers you grow. (See page 143 for more information.) You can remind yourself to wear your garden gloves by planting an herb garden in the shape of your hand, with a different herb growing along each finger.

Working in the garden our feet are usually covered by rubber boots or tennis shoes. Using foot powders, such as the recipe for Calendula Foot Powder on page 154, will keep them dry and comfortable. If you happen to suffer from a foot odor problem try soaking your feet in black tea (see page 154). Tea is naturally astringent and deodorizing. This old-fashioned remedy really works!

Footbaths and foot soaks are wonderful ways to relax and refresh your feet after a long day. Try the Alfalfa Mint Footbath on page 152 when you feel fatigued and your whole body will feel refreshed and alive.

For fun you may also want to try mehndi. This ancient form of body adornment is a current fashion trend and many beauty salons are painting intricate designs on the hands and feet of their clients. These temporary tattoos are made with ground henna leaves and are easy to apply at home (see page 141).

Whether it's a foot soak, cream, or mehndi treatment, always start with clean hands and feet when using these natural products. Store your products in clean containers and keep them in a cool, dark, dry place. When you are finished with a nail or foot bath, discard your bathwater. These treatments are meant to be made fresh each time and should not be reused.

Pamper your hardworking hands and feet!

GARDEN MANICURE

Many people consider manicures an indulgence or vanity treatment for fancy nails. This just isn't so. Proper hand care is important for everyone, especially hands that have been busy in the garden. I like to set aside an hour once a week for my hands, and treat them to a bit of pampering. I find a manicure is even more enjoyable when shared with a spouse or friend.

Steps to follow for beautiful hands:

1. If you wear nail polish, remove all traces of it.

2. Put some fresh flower petals in warm water and soak your hands for 10 minutes. You may also use the recipe on page 139 for Elm Leaf Nail Solution, which helps soften your cuticles. Use a gentle nail brush and clean under each nail.

3. Massage a rich hand cream into your hands and cuticles. Try the recipe for Marigold Hand Cream on page 137. Gently push back your cuticles with a cotton-tipped orange stick. *Never cut your cuticles.*

4. Using a paper emery board, file your nails into squared-off ovals. This shape is more attractive and stronger than that of a sharp point or one that's straight across. It will also mean your nails will break less often. Always keep all of your nails the same length.

5. Make a hand mask, using your favorite facial mask recipe. I prefer to use sour cream with a bit of honey and fresh herbs. Leave the mask on your hands for 15–20 minutes.

(continued)

6. Rinse off all of the mask with warm water, followed by cool water.

7. Massage a rich hand cream into your hands. Work from the base of your palm to your fingertips, one finger at a time. Wrap your hands in plastic wrap and let sit for 15–20 minutes. Unwrap your hands and remove any excess cream from them.

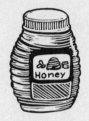

Marigold Hand Cream

This rich cream will nourish and protect your hands. A good hand cream can keep your skin smooth and supple by protecting it from moisture loss, preventing dirt from getting into the skin, and restoring the balance of acidity that can be upset by harsh, alkaline soaps. I like to use it before and after gardening or other household tasks to keep my hands looking and feeling lovely.

3 tablespoons fresh marigold petals
½ cup boiling water
⅛ teaspoon borax powder
1 tablespoon grated beeswax
1 tablespoon cocoa butter
½ cup almond oil

Place the fresh petals in a ceramic dish and gently crush them to release the plant juices. Pour the boiling water over the petals and let sit until cool, about 20 minutes. Strain and stir the borax into the petal liquid. Keep stirring until the borax is completely dissolved. In another heat-resistant pan or bowl mix together the beeswax, cocoa butter, and almond oil. Gently warm the mixture in a water bath or microwave until the beeswax and cocoa butter are melted. (The water bath is made by filling a pan with an inch of water and placing a glass jar containing the beeswax and cocoa butter in the pan.) Gradually stir in the borax and marigold flower infusion. Keep heating the mixture and stirring until well blended. You may also pour the entire mixture into a blender and blend on Medium until well mixed. Let the mixture cool completely. You may need to give it one more good mixing before using. Pour into a clean container with a tight-fitting lid.

Garden Note: When making fresh flower arrangements, especially those containing marigolds, try this "water" for long-lasting blooms: Mix together one quart water, two tablespoons sugar, and one tablespoon salt. Fill your vase and add fresh flowers.

Yield: 8 ounces

Prehistoric Nail Strengthener

1 teaspoon fresh horsetail stems,
  chopped
½ cup boiling water
1 teaspoon pure honey

Horsetail is an herb that can be traced back to prehistoric times. It grew and flourished some 200 million years ago at the same time the dinosaurs roamed the earth. The stems have a high silica content and are rich in minerals and natural salts. The hollow stems absorb important minerals such as gold, iron, magnesium, and potassium from the soil. A solution made from these stems can help strengthen your hair and nails.

Place the horsetail stems in a glass or ceramic dish. Pour the boiling water over them and let sit for 30 minutes. Strain off the stems and discard. Add the honey and stir well. Let this solution sit for a few days. Pour into a clean bottle with a tight-fitting lid. To use: Brush the solution over your nails using a clean cotton swab or small brush, and let dry. Do this every day for 10–14 days and you should see an improvement in the condition of your nails. You may also use this solution to soak your nails in when giving yourself a manicure.

Garden Note: Many people think of horsetail as a pesky weed because it grows profusely and once it is established it is hard to remove. It can be found growing along roadsides and in the woods. If you decide to grow it in your yard, do so in a container.

Yield: 4 ounces

Elm Leaf Nail Solution

Elm trees are a common neighborhood tree. They are magnificent shade trees that can cover an entire yard, which is not surprising, considering that they are fast growers and survive in a variety of soil conditions. Their green leaves make a moisturizing nail bath for dry, brittle nails.

1 cup fresh elm leaves, washed and chopped
2 cups boiling water
⅛ teaspoon vitamin E oil

Place the leaves in a glass or ceramic bowl and pour the boiling water over them. Cover the mixture and let sit until completely cool. Discard the leaves and stir in the vitamin E oil. Pour this solution into a clean container. To use: Soak your nails in this nail solution for 5–10 minutes daily. You may also brush the solution onto clean, dry nails, but do not rinse.

Garden Note: Use pruned tree branches as garden stakes to support your plants. They are natural and blend right into your flower beds.

Yield: 12 ounces

Hawaiian Cuticle Softener

If you have ever visited the Hawaiian islands then you have seen the acres and acres of fresh pineapples growing there. I love the look of these plants, which have dense, spiny leaves and a pineapple fruit sitting at their center. These fruits contain an active enzyme called bromelain. It is effective in softening rough, dry skin. It can also be drying, so to counteract this I have added an egg yolk to this recipe.

1 egg yolk
2 tablespoons fresh pineapple juice

Mix together the egg yolk and pineapple juice and stir well. To use: Spread this mixture on your cuticles and let it sit for 5 minutes. Using a cotton-covered orange stick or cotton swab, gently push back the softened cuticle skin against your nail bed. Never cut your cuticles as this could damage them. Rinse with warm water to remove the mixture. Then massage some coconut oil or rich hand cream into your hands. Discard any leftover product.

Garden Note: You can try to grow your own pineapple plant indoors. Cut off the top from a fresh pineapple and place it in a shallow dish of water. When roots appear, plant it in a pot filled with rich soil. Keep your plant in a sunny, warm location. If you are lucky, a new pineapple will grow in about two years.

Yield: 1 ounce, enough for one treatment

Jojoba Bean Cuticle Cream

2 tablespoons sunflower oil
2 tablespoons jojoba oil
1 teaspoon anhydrous lanolin or
    lanolin cream
½ teaspoon coconut oil

This is a rich cuticle cream made with jojoba bean oil that you can use when giving yourself a manicure. Massage it into your cuticles to condition them and increase your nails' circulation. Cuticles protect your nails, so it is important never to cut them. Instead, you should gently push them back with a clean cotton swab or cotton-wrapped orange stick. Jojoba bean oil can be found at any natural food store.

Combine the ingredients in an oven-proof glass container and heat gently in a double boiler or a microwave. When all the ingredients have melted, pour the mixture into a clean container. Cool completely before using. To use: Massage a small amount of the cream into each cuticle.

Garden Note: To keep your hands looking their best always massage them with a rich hand cream before putting on your garden gloves.

Yield: 2 ounces

Mehndi

If you ever toyed with the idea of getting a tattoo or are looking for a new type of temporary body adornment, then mehndi, the ancient practice of dying the skin with henna, may be for you. Traditionally, it is used in India to embellish the hands of brides before their wedding. Today the delicate filigree designs have become a fashion statement that many salons offer. Unlike traditional tattoos, mehndi is temporary (lasting only a few weeks), safe, and natural. The designs are drawn on top of the skin using a paste made from crushed henna leaves. This gives the designs a soft color. After reading about this practice, my daughters and I all painted small tattoos on our feet. It was fun, easy, and lasted about a month. For our mehndi day I purchased ground henna leaves—you can choose powder too—at my natural food store. Many pharmacies also carry henna powder; look for it in the hair care section.

¼ cup henna powder, finely sifted (make sure you remove large stems and leaves)

¼ cup boiling water

2 tea bags (orange pekoe or black tea works best)

Fresh lemon juice

Pour the boiling water over the tea bags to make a strong tea. Let steep for at least an hour. Place your sifted henna in a glass or ceramic bowl. Slowly add the tea until you have a smooth creamy paste (you may not use it all). Let this mixture sit for several hours, or even overnight, to let the color come out of the henna. If the mixture seems too dry, add a bit more water and stir well. Decide on your design and where you want it to go. Make sure your skin is clean. Natural oils and lotions can prevent the henna from working. I would start with a simple, small design.

To paint with your henna paste: Place it in a pastry bag or a plastic bag with one corner snipped off, or use a small brush. What you use for application will depend on your design. Write with the henna wherever you wish the design to appear. It will stain, so be careful. Once you have finished your design, let the henna dry on your skin, dabbing it every now and then with a slice of lemon. The skin absorbs the henna dye slowly, so keeping it moist will help, for the longer it sits on your skin the darker the design will be. Some people cover their designs and leave the henna on overnight. I have let mine sit for 2 to 3 hours and was satisfied with the color. Rinse off the henna with warm water and rub the design with more lemon juice. Voila! Your design will darken a bit more as the lemon juice dries. Mehndi should last for several weeks to a month, depending upon where you made your design on your body and how often it is washed.

Garden Note: Henna plants are found in North Africa and the Middle East. These large shrubs can grow up to twenty feet high and enjoy hot weather with full sun. Their leaves and stems have been used as a beauty ingredient since ancient times. Henna can be used to dye and condition the hair, strengthen nails, and decorate the body.

Yield: 2 ounces

Green Thumb Hand Cream

3 tablespoons grated beeswax
½ cup dark sesame oil
1 tablespoon coconut oil
1 teaspoon honey
2 tablespoons strong calendula tea
2–3 drops essential oil of lavender
⅛ teaspoon baking soda

Green thumbs and rough dry hands no longer need to be the result of a day spent gardening. It is possible to grow and tend healthy plants and flowers without destroying your hands. Use this rich cream before and after a day spent planting, weeding, and pruning. It will keep your hands soft and full of moisture. I like to massage it into my hands before putting on my gardening gloves. The dark sesame oil acts as a mild sunscreen, and the scent of lavender is a natural insect repellent.

Combine all ingredients in a glass, heat-resistant container or double boiler. Heat in the microwave or over medium heat on the stove until all the wax and oils are melted (do not boil), stirring well. Pour the melted mixture into a container or jar and allow to cool completely. Stir again when the mixture has cooled.

Yield: 4 ounces

Garden Glove Selection

The best hand care advice I can give you for working in your garden is to apply a good sunscreen and always wear a pair of garden gloves. Your hands are your most important garden tool and they deserve proper protection. Walk the glove aisle of your local garden or hardware shop and you will be amazed at the number of different glove styles available. Selecting the right glove for the job will keep your hands looking and feeling wonderful. Your gloves should fit snugly and be easy to put on and take off. When I shop for a new pair of gloves I look for fit, durability, and design. I also like gloves that are easy to care for. There are three main types of gloves: cotton, rubber, and leather:

Cotton: These gloves are lightweight and comfortable. In hot weather they provide extra comfort by absorbing perspiration. They are also washable. Cotton gloves are inexpensive (a few dollars a pair), so it is possible to purchase more than one pair at a time (helpful if one pair is in the wash or you garden both inside and out). They do, however, wear out faster than other glove types and can tear or stretch. They are also unsuited for extremely wet jobs, as they get soggy and often you will end up taking them off—which defeats their purpose. For light weeding of dry earth and container planting they are perfect.

Rubber: These provide the best protection from wetness, chemicals, and poisonous plants. They are a good choice if you have sensitive skin and do not want to develop a rash from a particular plant. They are good for extremely wet jobs because they keep your hands dry. Rubber gloves come in various thicknesses and sizes—there are even gauntlet-style gloves for water gardening. I like to purchase disposable (surgical-style) gloves that may be worn alone or under cotton gloves. These are fairly inexpensive and can often be purchased in bulk (50–100 at a time). Because they are thinner they allow me to handle small seeds and delicate plants. The one negative may be that they do not allow for air circulation around your hands, and in hot weather they hold in moisture which could cause your hands to chap. If this becomes a problem, remove your gloves often and sprinkle a bit of cornstarch or body powder inside them. A newer style I have seen combines the comfort of cotton with the protection of rubber. These gloves are cotton based, with the fingers and palms covered in latex.

Leather: These gloves are similar to cotton in use but much more durable and sturdy. They are more expensive than the cotton varieties, but a good pair of leather gloves can last several gardening seasons. Many are hand-washable using a mild soap and left to air-dry. Cowhide is the toughest and good to wear when you are using heavy equipment, such as a rototiller. Pigskin is probably the most popular because it is softer and easily cleaned. Goatskin is the top of the line as far as softness goes, but it does not wear as well as the other two. For light weeding and use of hand tools, goatskin gloves are quite elegant and provide better dexterity than the heavier leathers. If you are working around prickly plants, such as roses, you may also want to purchase longer gloves that protect your forearms.

It is important that you choose a glove style that fits your gardening habits—that is, for container planting, power tool usage, pruning, or heavy weeding. So, think about how you spend your time in the garden before purchasing your gloves.

Garden-Stained Hands

Forget to wear your gloves? It is easy to do. I often find myself reaching down to rid the garden of a few pesky weeds and before I know it I have a huge pile of weeds and a pair of dirty, stained hands. Here is a simple tip that involves using fresh lemons or green tomatoes, both of which really work to clean and refresh your hands. Remember to moisturize well afterward, because this treatment can be drying to your skin.

Fresh lemons: Lemons are natural astringents and disinfectants that will leave your hands clean and fragrant. Cut a lemon in half and rub the fresh juice all over your hands. Leave the juice on your hands for 5 minutes, then rinse well with warm water.

Green tomatoes: Working around tomato plants can give the skin on your hands a yellow-green tint. Use a green tomato to remove these stains. Cut the fruit in half and rub the fresh juice all over your hands. Leave the juice on your hands for 5 minutes, then rinse well with warm water.

Yield: one treatment

Total Foot Care

The word pedicure *means "caring for the feet." Follow these steps for the ultimate in foot care. This is an intense treatment from which your whole body can benefit. Weekly pedicures are important to keep your feet looking and feeling happy and healthy. If the weather is right, perform the following steps out-doors under the warm sun:*

1. Soak your feet for 15–20 minutes in a warm foot-bath. Try the recipe for Juniper Berry Footbath on page 148. Use a nail brush and really clean under each toenail. Use a wet pumice stone or exfoliating scrub (try cornmeal, ground almonds, or clean beach sand) to gently rub away hard skin on your feet.

2. Trim your toenails after soaking them. It is easier to do and you will get a cleaner cut. Cut the nails straight across to avoid ingrown nails.

3. Apply a foot mask. Try the recipe for Happy Feet Mask on page 153. I also like to make a foot mask with some natural clay mixed with water and a few drops of eucalyptus oil. Wrap your feet in plastic wrap and elevate them for 15–20 minutes.

4. Rinse your feet well with warm water followed by cool.

5. Massage a rich cuticle cream (see page 139) into your toenails and gently push back the cuticles at the base of each nail. Never cut your cuticles; they play an important role in protecting your nails from infections.

6. Massage a light oil or cream (see page 137) into your feet and elevate them again for 15–20 minutes. If you are enjoying a pedicure in the evening, slip on some cotton socks and leave them on all night.

GIVE YOURSELF A FOOT MASSAGE

A soothing foot massage is something you can easily do for yourself. It is relaxing and beneficial to your whole body. The science of reflexology is based upon the belief that every part of your body is influenced by the massage of an associated place on the soles of your feet. Tension can be relieved, circulation increased, and total peace achieved simply by massaging your feet. Reflexology charts are available at many bookstores, natural food stores, and libraries if you want to learn more about it. Here is a basic foot massage sure to make you a believer in the soothing that foot attention provides. Go through all the steps on one foot and then do the other.

1. Sit where you are comfortable. Rotate each ankle clockwise and counterclockwise to loosen your muscles.

2. Warm some cream or massage oil in your palms then start to apply it at your toes, working toward your ankle in a circular motion.

3. Squeeze each toe gently, then work your fingers down each side. Move on to the sole of your foot, kneading your muscles and concentrating on any hard spots.

4. Complete the massage by working your fingers around the outside of the heel and ending at the center.

5. Repeat the massage with the other foot. When finished, gently shake your feet from side to side and then put both feet up and relax for 5–10 minutes.

Juniper Berry Footbath

¼ cup fresh juniper berries, crushed
¼ cup Epsom salts
1–2 tablespoons baking soda

All around my parents' home in Oregon are large western juniper trees. These evergreen trees produce small blue berries that can be used in making gin, flavoring cooking dishes, and creating refreshing baths and body oils. The fall is the best time to harvest fresh berries. You can gather and dry them to use in recipes all year long. You may also purchase dried berries at many natural food stores or gourmet food shops. Juniper berries are naturally antiseptic, making them well suited for a cleansing and refreshing footbath like this one.

Fill a large tub or bucket with warm water. Add the juniper berries, Epsom salts, and baking soda and stir well until the salts and soda have dissolved. Soak your feet in the fragrant water for 15–20 minutes. After your footbath, massage your feet with some natural oils or a rich foot cream.

Garden Note: If you are planting juniper trees in your yard make sure you plant a male and a female. You need both to produce berries. Male trees have yellow flowers at the tips of their shoots; female shoots are green.

Yield: 4 ounces, enough for one footbath

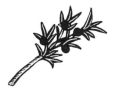

Garden boots are notorious for causing calluses and rough spots on your feet. To help soothe tired feet and remove rough skin spots it is best to soak your feet in a lukewarm bath of baking soda and vinegar. I also like to add a few of my favorite herbs, such as thyme and lavender, both of which are naturally antiseptic and comforting. After soaking for at least ten minutes, use a natural pumice stone or piece of terra-cotta to further smooth and remove calluses caused by stiff boots or shoes. To keep calluses from recurring wear double socks or cushioned inserts inside your boots and make sure boots fit properly.

Garden Boot Bath

2 quarts warm water
¼ cup baking soda
¼ cup herbal vinegar or plain white vinegar
1 tablespoon fresh lavender flowers and leaves
1 tablespoon fresh thyme leaves

Fill a large plastic pan or sink with warm water. Stir in the baking soda, vinegar, and fresh herbs. The water will fizz and bubble when the soda and vinegar combine. To use: Soak your feet for 15–20 minutes. Pat dry and massage them with a rich natural oil or foot cream.

Garden Note: I have a pair of boots outside my back door to slip into before going out into the garden. Footwear is a matter of personal preference. Just make sure your shoes have good arch support (important when using a shovel) and will keep your feet dry.

Garden Note: Display fresh herbs as if they were flowers. Just gather a bunch, snip off the ends, and immerse quickly in water. I use common containers such as glasses, jars, even teapots. They last longer than many flowers, and you will have fresh herbs ready to use in beauty recipes.

Yield: 64 ounces, enough for one footbath

River Stone Footbath

½ cup sea salt or Epsom salts
2 quarts cool water
Small river stones or marbles
1–2 drops camphor oil (optional)

If you have ever camped or hiked next to a river or small stream you know how refreshing it is just to sit along the shore and soak your feet. The pure, cold water is exhilarating. You find yourself picking up small pebbles and stones with your toes as they cool in the moving water. You can recreate this mountain foot spa in your own home. Place a few saved river stones inside this footbath for your feet to pick up and roll back and forth. This is actually an excellent foot exercise that stretches your muscles and relaxes your feet.

Fill a shallow tub or bucket with water. Pour in the salts and camphor oil and stir well until dissolved.

Place a collection of small stones or marbles in your bath container. Soak your feet for 15–20 minutes, gently rolling them back and forth over the stones. Occasionally pick up a stone with your toes and then release it; this action stretches and relaxes your feet.

Garden Note: Use special outdoor concrete paint to decorate your stepping-stones. This can be purchased at any hardware or paint store. Paint free-hand flowers and messages, or use stencils and masking tape for more uniform designs. You could try painting a walkway full of stripes, diamonds, stars, or polka dots. I once visited a delightful garden with bright daisies painted on round stepping-stones along with cheerful garden quotes. These were fun to walk on and very inspirational! You can also paint matching garden accessories such as watering cans, flowerpots, hose containers, and wheelbarrows.

Yield: 64 ounces, enough for one footbath

Alfalfa Mint Footbath

Alfalfa is a member of the soybean (peanut) family. Arabs discovered it two thousand years ago and called it al-fal-fa, which translates to "father of all foods." Combined with cooling herbs, such as mint and thyme, it makes an energizing footbath. This soak, followed by a simple foot massage using a natural oil such as grapeseed or sunflower, will do wonders for tired overworked feet. You may also use fresh alfalfa and herbs in this recipe by simply doubling the amounts called for.

1 gallon hot water
2 tablespoons Epsom salts
2 tablespoons dried alfalfa leaves
1 tablespoon dried mint leaves
1 tablespoon dried thyme leaves

Place the dried or fresh herbs inside a tea ball or square of cheesecloth. Fill your footbath with the hot water and pour in the Epsom salts. Float your herbal bundle in the water and let it steep until the water is cool enough for your feet. To use: Soak your feet in the soft, fragrant water for 15–20 minutes. Pat your skin dry and massage a rich natural oil into your feet.

Yield: 128 ounces, enough for one footbath

PUMICE STONES

Natural pumice stones are actually bits of super-cooled volcanic lava. They have been used for ages to remove dead skin and calluses from the feet. If you do not live in a volcanic region where you may find pumice stone, you may purchase these natural rocks at most pharmacy and natural food stores.

Pumice stones always work best when wet. Soak the stone for 3–5 minutes. Immerse feet in soapy water for 10 minutes; then slather on a rich cream and rub the stone over your feet in a circular motion.

Natural stones are hard to sterilize, so never share your stone with others and allow it to air-dry completely between uses. Better yet, discard the stone every two to three months and replace with a fresh, clean stone. You may also create a pumice powder by crushing your stone with a hammer. This can be added to foot creams and lotions to help exfoliate rough skin.

Happy Feet Mask

Steve Martin used to have a comedy routine in the '70s that always made me laugh out loud. His feet were so happy that he could not control them. It was as if they had a mind of their own as they danced and carried him all around the stage. This foot mask made with fresh ingredients should make your feet equally happy and carefree. It may even make them want to dance!

2 teaspoons chopped fresh mint leaves
2 tablespoons fresh pineapple juice
1 teaspoon chopped fresh basil leaves
2 teaspoons chopped fresh rosemary leaves
1–2 tablespoons plain yogurt

Place all the ingredients in a blender or food processor and mix well until you have a thick cream. To use: Spread the foot mask on clean feet, massaging it into your skin. Pay special attention to classic rough skin areas such as heels and toe pads. Wrap your feet in plastic wrap or cover them with thick cotton socks. Let the mask remain on your feet 15–20 minutes. Rinse well with cool water. Your feet should be very happy!

Garden Note: Old panty hose can be cut up in strips and used to tie up delicate plants. The soft material is strong but will not cut into growing plants.

Yield: 2 ounces, enough for one foot mask

FRIENDLY FERNS

If you are hiking in the woods or along a country road and your feet begin to hurt, this idea should help ease the soreness. Soothe your feet with fresh fern leaves. Cut off a few fronds and place them inside your boots. They will provide a quick and refreshing cushion for your tired feet. Just remember to clean out your boots when you get home. You do not want the ferns' fronds to dry out or decompose inside your boots after they are no longer needed.

Calendula Foot Powder

¼ cup cornstarch or rice flour
2 tablespoons baking soda
1 tablespoon finely ground, dried
    calendula petals
1–2 drops essential oil of geranium

Calendula, or "pot marigolds," have bright orange-yellow flowers that bloom profusely from spring to fall. Sometimes, given the right growing conditions, they will grow year-round. Old-time gardeners will tell you that they usually flower on the first day of each month. This may be the reasoning behind the botanical name, taken from the Latin calends, or "calendar." Dried flower petals have antibacterial properties and combined with baking soda make a soothing, deodorizing foot powder.

Place all the ingredients in a dry jar or resealable plastic bag and shake well to mix. Pour the powder into a clean, dry container. To use: Sprinkle the powder on clean, dry feet and gently massage into the skin, especially between the toes.

Garden Note: Whenever I am cleaning up my calendula patch by dead-heading the flowers, I easily reseed it by scattering the dried seeds from the old flower heads over the soil. A light raking with a hand fork keeps my flower plot growing continuously with new plants.

Yield: 3 ounces

Foot Odor Cure

2 cups boiling water
2 black tea bags
2 quarts of cool water

After a day spent in garden boots your feet may not smell as good as your precious flowers. To sweeten your feet or cure a foot odor problem try a foot soak in natural tea. Soaking your feet in black tea will help reduce foot odor because tea is naturally astringent. It can help reduce the amount of perspiration your feet produce, which can add up to ½ cup in a day! The tannic acid in the tea changes your skin's pH level, making it unfriendly to odor-causing bacteria. Keeping your feet moisturized will also help prevent dry skin and keep bacteria levels down. So, after this footbath, use a rich foot cream or lotion.

Make a very strong tea by steeping the two tea bags in the boiling water for at least 15 minutes. Fill a large bowl or plastic pan with the cool water and stir in the tea solution. Soak your feet for 20–30 minutes. Repeat this treatment every day for about a week. You should notice a decrease in foot odor.

Garden Note: Wellington boots (knee-length rubber boots) are well suited for garden use. They are sturdy, light, and slip on easily. They can also be rinsed off with the garden hose. Keep your boots and feet dry and smelling fresh by sprinkling some cornstarch or foot powder inside them.

Yield: 80 ounces, enough for one footbath

GARDENER'S GIFT BASKET

In the spring when garden activities begin to pick up, give your friends a basket full of pampering products and tools for their hard-working hands and feet. This thoughtful gift will keep them looking and feeling great. Don't forget to put together one for yourself as well! Here are a few suggestions for filling up your container:

- Green Thumb Hand Cream, see page 142
- New pair of garden gloves
- Nail brush
- Alfalfa Mint Footbath, see page 151
- New pumice stone
- Calendula Foot Powder, see page 154
- Beauty plant seed packets such as sunflower, loofah, cucumber, or favorite herbs

Homemade Soap

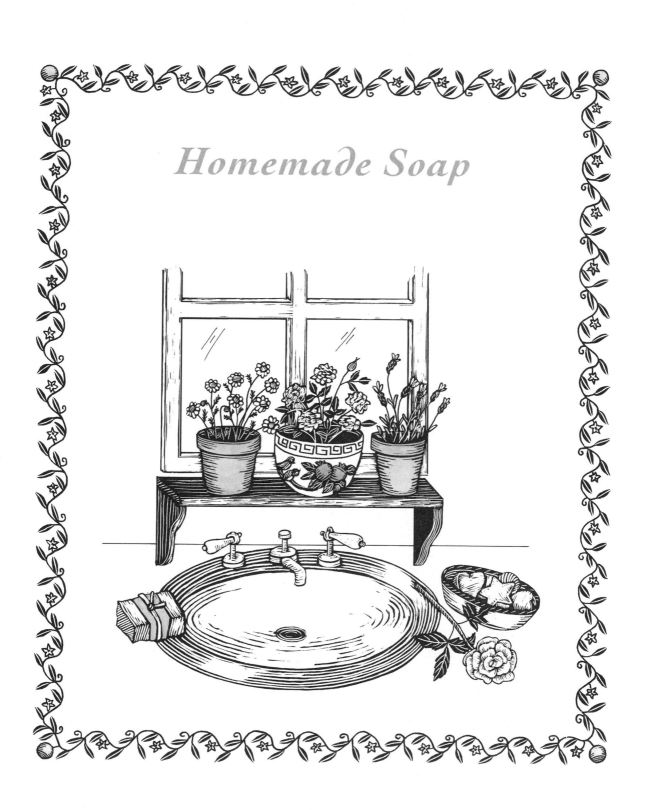

*H*omemade soap is a pioneer necessity that has become a modern-day cottage industry phenomenon. It seems everyone is getting into the soap business, from fashion designers to homemakers—and you can too!

Soap is the oldest of all cleaning products. It dates back to 1000 B.C. where it was discovered in Rome on Sapo Hill. An ancient story tells of a woman rinsing her clothes in the river at the base of a hill. Above the river animals had been recently sacrificed. The rendered animal fat soaked through the wood ashes (lye) creating a soapy mud, which in turn got her clothes incredibly clean.

Today we still use the same fundamental ingredients (fat and lye) with several new twists and improvements. The use of natural vegetable oils, such as olive, palm, and coconut, has become popular. These natural oils have replaced animal products in many commercial soaps. Bars containing essential oils and dried botanicals are easy to find and wonderful to use. In fact, soap is one of your best beauty buys. A new bar is a welcome treat that can bring a bit of luxury to an everyday routine.

Soap making is an art form. It is also a simple process that anyone can master. It does, however, take an attention to detail, practice, and a bit of patience. I can tell you that my first bar of soap was anything but white and fluffy. It also took a bit of persuasion to get my family to use it. Today, several batches of soap later, I can now turn out a decent bar, suitable for gift-giving. It is also very rewarding to use your own soap—nothing smells or feels quite as clean.

Soap has three main ingredients: water, lye, and fat. Lye is also known as sodium hydroxide or caustic soda. Pioneers produced lye solutions by pouring water through wood ashes. I purchase lye granules at the hardware store (it is used as a drain opener). Craft stores, soap-making supply catalogs, and chemical supply shops also sell it. Fat can be derived from a number of sources. I like to use pure vegetable fats and oils in my recipes. Many old-fashioned soap recipes call for animal products, such as tallow and lard. I do not find these as appealing as vegetable oils, but you can choose to use them if you like.

"Saponification" is the name given the chemical process for making soap. The key to its success is temperature. The lye, mixed with cold water, must cool down to a certain temperature (when lye is mixed with water, the tem-

---

BASIC SOAP-MAKING RULES

1. Always wear rubber gloves and protective clothing: long-sleeved shirts, long pants, and shoes.

2. Work in a well-ventilated area.

3. Keep some vinegar nearby to rub on your skin. If lye gets on it, the vinegar will neutralize it. *Always handle lye with extreme caution—it can cause severe burns.*

4. Always use cold water when mixing the lye solution.

5. Avoid all distractions. Soap making requires your full attention. (Unplug the phone if you must.)

6. Use a thermometer to monitor fat/oil and lye temperatures.

7. Always pour the lye solution into the fat or oil mixture, not the other way around.

---

perature rises to over 200 degrees Fahrenheit), and the fat/oils must be heated up to a certain temperature. When the temperatures are right, the oil is saponified into soap by the lye. This process can take hours or even days; good soap is best if aged for at least a month.

The recipes in this section are ones for basic soaps to help you get started in the art of soap making. I suggest reading through each recipe several times before starting. Make sure you have everything you need before beginning. Soap making requires some extra kitchen equipment that is unnecessary for most other recipes. Use old pans and jars, since they could get ruined during the process. Secondhand shops and garage sales are excellent sources for soap-making pans and molds.

Here is the list of equipment that I use:

> A pair of rubber gloves—to protect your hands.
>
> Candy thermometer (two, if you have them)—one for the oil temperature and one for the lye temperature. In soap making the right temperature is extremely important.
>
> Large enamel, glass, or steel pan (do not use aluminum)—to cook your soap in.
>
> Large glass jar with lid (punch two holes, opposite each other, in the lid with an ice-pick—to dissolve your lye in. Place the lid on the jar when pouring the lye into your oils.
>
> Wooden spoons—for stirring.
>
> Cardboard boxes and old muffin tins—for soap molds.

Your finished soaps will last longer in a warm, dry location. After using a bar of soap always place it in a soap dish where it can dry out between uses.

Have fun making soap the old-fashioned way, using just a few simple natural ingredients!

Basic Vegetable Soap

½ cup olive oil
½ cup coconut oil
1 cup vegetable shortening
½ cup lye granules
2 cups cold distilled water

This is a good recipe to start with. After you have mastered it you may want to try some variations by adding color, scent, and texture to your soaps. I like to use vegetable shortening, olive oil, and coconut oil. Combining these three fats produces a fine, soft soap with a creamy lather.

Mix the lye with the cold water in your glass jar. I like to do this the night before, because it takes a while for the solution to cool. It is always easier to raise the lye temperature before beginning than to wait for it to cool. (It will need to be at 75°F during soap making.)

Place the oils in a large saucepan; gently heat until melted and at a temperature of 85°F. Bring the lye solution up to the desired temperature of 75°F; this can be done by placing the jar in a pan of warm water.

With your two-holed lid on the lye jar, slowly pour the lye solution into the oil mixture in a thin, steady stream, with slow, even stirring. You should not be applying any heat to the mixture at this time. Continue stirring until you have a thick pudding-like texture. This should take about 10–20 minutes. Note: If the soap mixture does not become thick within 30 minutes, and there is a greasy layer on top, it may be too warm. Keep stirring.

Pour the thickened soap mixture into oiled molds. Cover and wrap your mold in an old towel or blanket to keep it warm and prevent the mixture from separating. When the soap is set, remove from the molds and cut into bars. You may also want to trim your soaps with a sharp paring knife. Allow the soap to age for at least 2 weeks in a dry place.

Variations to try:

*I*t is easy to add scent, color, or texture to your soaps. After saponification—when your soap is thick and pudding-like— add essential oils, dried herbs, flowers, cornmeal, or ground nuts to your mixture and stir well using 5–6 drops of essential oil and 1–2 tablespoons of any dried materials. Here are a few suggestions to try:

Cleansing almond and oatmeal: almond fragrance oil, ground almonds, and ground oatmeal.

Relaxing lavender: lavender essential oil and dried lavender flowers.

Romantic rose spice: cinnamon essential oil, ground cinnamon, and dried rosebuds.

Garden Note: Install an outdoor soap dish near your garden hose. Keep a bar of soap there for easy, convenient garden cleanups.

Yield: 12 2-ounce bars (depending on the size mold you use)

*A*vocado oil is a good choice for people with dry or sensitive skin because it is so mild. It is obtained from the fruit's buttery pulp and is valuable in soap making because it contains a high percentage of unsaponifiable oil (oil that will not react with the lye to form soap). Because of this it makes a very rich, moisturizing soap. Avocado oil can be purchased at most grocery stores in the cooking oil section.

Mix the lye with the cold water in your glass jar. I like to do this the night before, because it takes a while for

Avocado Oil Soap

½ cup olive oil
½ cup avocado oil
¼ cup cocoa butter
1 cup coconut oil
½ cup lye granules
2 cups cold distilled water

the solution to cool. It is always easier to raise the lye temperature before beginning than to wait for it to cool. (It will need to be at 75°F during soap making.)

Place the oils and cocoa butter in a large saucepan. Gently heat the oils until melted and at a temperature of 85°F. Bring the lye solution up to the desired temperature of 75°F. This can be done by placing the jar in a pan of warm water.

With your two-holed lid on the lye jar, slowly pour the lye solution into the oil mixture in a thin, steady stream, with slow, even stirring. You should not be applying any heat to the mixture at this time. Continue stirring until you have a thick pudding-like texture. This should take 10–20 minutes. Note: If the soap mixture does not become thick within 30 minutes, and there is a greasy layer on top, it may be too warm. Keep stirring.

Pour the thickened soap mixture into oiled molds. Cover and wrap your mold in an old towel or blanket to keep it warm and prevent the mixture from separating. When the soap is set, remove from the molds and cut into bars. You may also want to trim your soaps with a sharp paring knife. Allow the soap to age for at least 2 weeks in a dry place.

Garden Note: I am told by many of my country friends that placing bars of soap around your garden will keep away hungry, plant-destroying deer.

Yield: 12 2-ounce bars (depending on the size mold you use)

Coffee Bar

I have a habit of drinking my morning coffee in the shower. This mixing of cleansing and body wake-up has become a part of my morning routine. In Europe caffeine has become an ingredient in creams, lotions, and soaps. It is believed to stimulate the body and help rid it of cellulite. I doubt simply applying coffee topically can break down body fat and firm muscles—but it does make the products smell delicious. By using strong coffee as part of the liquid in this recipe you obtain a soap with a warm color and mild scent—perfect for morning showers.

½ cup almond oil
½ cup coconut oil
1 cup vegetable shortening
½ cup lye granules
1 cup cold distilled water
1 cup cold strong-brewed coffee

Mix the lye with the cold water and coffee in your glass jar. I like to do this the night before, because it takes a while for the solution to cool. It is always easier to raise the lye temperature before beginning than to wait for it to cool. (It will need to be at 75°F during soap making.)

Place the oils in a large saucepan. Gently heat the oils until melted and at a temperature of 85°F. Bring the lye solution up to the desired temperature of 75°F. This can be done by placing the jar in a pan of warm water.

With your two-holed lid on the lye jar, slowly pour the lye solution into the oil mixture, in a thin, steady stream with slow, even stirring. You should not be applying any heat to the mixture at this time. Continue stirring until you have a thick pudding-like texture. This should take about 10–20 minutes. Note: If the soap mixture does not become thick within 30 minutes, and there is a greasy layer on top, it may be too warm. Keep stirring.

Pour the thickened soap mixture into oiled molds. Cover and wrap your mold in an old towel or blanket to keep it warm and prevent the mixture from separating. When the soap is set, remove from the molds and cut into bars. You may also want to trim your soaps using a sharp paring knife. Allow the soap to age for at least 2 weeks in a dry place.

Variation:

For a bit of texture, add a tablespoon or two of ground coffee beans to your soap mixture before pouring it into the molds.

Garden Note: Plants love coffee. My daughter did her science experiment this year by watering grass seed with different liquids. The grass that got the coffee grew faster and thicker. You may also add your used tea bags and coffee grounds to the ground beneath acid-loving plants such as camellias and rhododendrons.

Yield: 12 2-ounce bars (depending on the size mold you use)

Easy Molded Soaps

6 cups grated soap
⅓ cup water
¼ cup dried lavender, ground almonds, or ground oatmeal
Essential oils, your choice (optional)

If you want the look of homemade soaps but are not sure you want to get involved in the whole lye/fat process, this easy recipe is for you. You can create pleasing natural soaps. Simply melt down purchased bars of glycerine, castile, or other pure soaps. Adding natural scents and ingredients makes them unique and gives them that homemade touch. This is also a great way to recycle old bars and soap slivers. You will need cookie cutters, cookie sheets or a large baking pan, some aluminum foil, and a double boiler.

Prepare your molds by oiling the cookie cutters and covering one side with some aluminum foil. Place them on a cookie sheet.

Combine the soap and water in a double boiler and melt over medium heat, stirring—do not boil.

Add your fragrance—oil-based scents work best. Some perfumes and colognes may separate your mixture. Add texture with dried herbs, flowers, nuts, and grains.

Working quickly, fill your molds generously. After your soap has cooled you may trim off any excess with a sharp knife.

When the soap is cool, remove from the molds and air-dry for at least 24 hours.

Yield: 14 ounces

Fresh-as-a-Daisy Soap

White and yellow daisies have always symbolized the ultimate in freshness. Chamomile plants have their own petite flower or daisy that has a fresh apple-like scent and bright appearance. They also have anti-inflammatory properties, making them well-suited for calming sensitive skin. I like to add them to molded soaps. Try placing a fresh flower at the bottom of each mold for a decorative touch.

2 bars of grated glycerine soap
1 tablespoon cocoa butter
1 tablespoon water
2 tablespoons chamomile flowers, fresh or dried

In a double boiler place the soap, cocoa butter, and water. Gently heat until the soap and cocoa butter are melted and you have a thick pudding-like mixture. Stir in the chamomile flowers and spoon the mixture into oiled molds. Let the soaps harden, then remove from the molds. You may trim your soaps using a sharp knife.

Yield: 8 ounces, 2–3 bars of soap

Loofah Soap

2 bars of pure natural soap, such as
   castile or coconut oil
2 tablespoons vegetable glycerine
1 tablespoon water
4 slices dried loofah sponge, ½-inch
   thick

These are gentle scrubbing bars that are useful in cleaning your hands after a day of gardening. You can also use them to cleanse your whole body. The natural loofah sponge helps exfoliate dead skin cells and surface impurities, leaving your skin clean, soft, and smooth. Do not use this soap to wash your face, as it may be too harsh. I use a serrated bread knife to slice the dried loofah gourd.

Place the loofah slices on an oiled cookie sheet. In a double boiler gently heat the soap, glycerine, and water until you have a thick mixture and all the soap is melted. Spoon the melted soap inside your loofah slices and allow it to harden. Trim your soaps with a sharp knife. To use: Use as you would a loofah sponge or any scrubbing bar of soap. Avoid broken skin or sensitive areas.

Yield: 8 ounces, 3–4 bars of soap

Enjoy Your Soaps!

Here are several ways to use, decorate, give, and savor your home-made creations:

- Wrap your soap bars in natural fabrics, such as cotton, linen, or silk, like you would a present. Tie with a pretty ribbon or scrap of raffia.

- Draw decorative labels for your soaps on a strip of paper (or use your computer). Wrap a strip around the bar and set with a drop of glue. Corrugated cardboard also makes a nice band for your soaps.

- Make liquid shower soaps: Dissolve equal parts grated soap in water. Add more scent if you wish.

- Carve your soap bars into interesting shapes or put catchy words and phrases on them.

- Mold a giant soap loaf and slice off a piece before bathing.

- For children of all ages, place small plastic objects inside the bars. These will appear as you use the soap. This works well with glycerine soaps.

- Sew scrubbing bars: Stitch a bar of soap inside a wash-cloth.

- Create your own soap on a rope. Mold your soap around a piece of cotton cord. This is handy in the shower!

- Use candy molds to create small, pretty guest soaps.

Bath Products

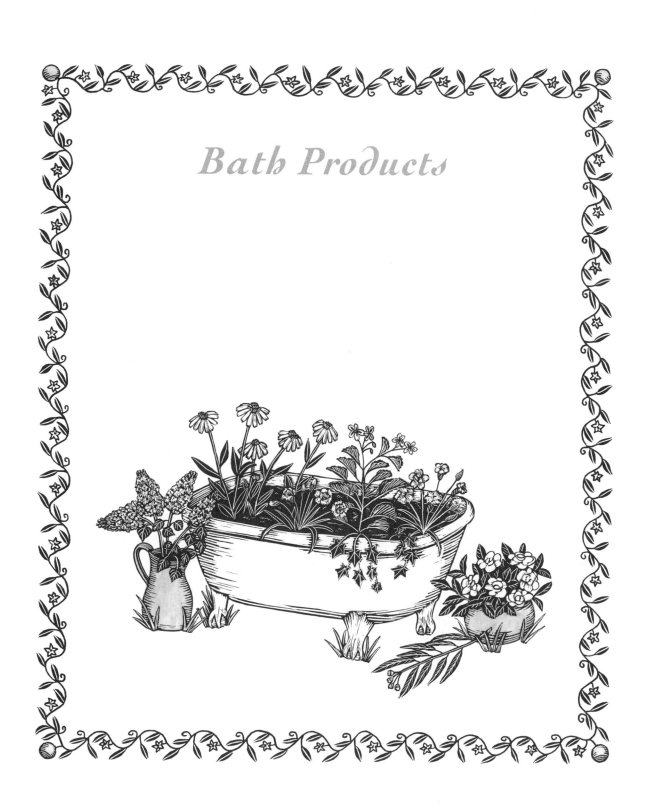

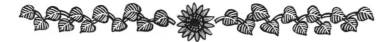

*T*he other day I had one of those nonstop, super-busy days. I'm sure you know the kind—in which every project and family member needs your attention and there just doesn't seem to be enough time for a moment to yourself. Usually on a day like this I go out in the garden and do some weeding to give myself some personal time and still be productive. But in this particular instance I didn't even have time for that. So, after tucking my daughters into bed and leaving my husband content watching his nightly business programs, I took some of my own advice: I took a bath! Not the basic get in, get clean, and get out type of washing, but an indulgent, luxurious *real* bath. I lit candles, made a pot of herbal tea, and read a favorite book. I filled my tea ball with some fragrant Tub Tea (see page 179) and luxuriated in the scented water. My crazy day and all its tensions and decisions went right down the drain with the bathwater. I emerged renewed, calm, and collected. In fact, my husband even looked up from the television to see my refreshed expression and asked what had happened. "The power of the bath," was my reply. A bath, something so simple to do, and so often overlooked as the stress-relieving rejuvenator that it is.

My own personal bathing revelation is really not that unusual. I recently read that 46 percent of American women say that their favorite method of escape and relaxation is to take a bath. People have used water for centuries to heal, cleanse, and relax the body. Hydrotherapy, as it is often called, is an ancient practice. Hippocrates, the father of modern medicine, praised the use of water and its benefits. Throughout history people have enjoyed taking a bath. Famous women and figures of legend such as Venus, Marie Antoinette, Mary Queen of Scots, and Cleopatra all attributed their great beauty to bathing rituals. Roman men solved problems and discussed current affairs in their communal baths. Is it any surprise that legendary idea man Ben Franklin is responsible for importing the first formal bathtub to America from France? It was made of copper and had a small furnace for heating the water under it. This was historic, as it enabled bathing to become private. No longer would it need to be done in the kitchen, where the water was traditionally heated; it could be moved to its own room.

Today the bathroom is one of the most important areas of the house. The degree to which this is true became apparent to me recently when my husband and I remodeled our own bathroom. The selection of fixtures and materials was almost overwhelming. The products offered today for the bath range from the functional to the fantastic. Bathing accessories are just as impressive, with brushes, sponges, compact discs, candles, tub toys, and designer towels being sold in boutiques, department stores, and specialty catalogs. Today bath products are the largest segment of the cosmetic market. The bath has become big business!

In this section you will find some of my favorite botanical bath and shower products inspired by the garden. I have included recipes for bringing a bit of the outdoors into your bath by creating indulgent botanical bath products. If you are feeling a bit daring, try the reverse and take the indoors out by showering or bathing outdoors (see page 204). I think this is the ultimate way to enjoy nature!

Follow the instructions on page 31 and fill large terra-cotta planters full of bath herbs and flowers or plant them in an old tub or sink and make it the focal point of your garden.

Bath products are easy and simple to create. Floral and herbal bath oils are some of the most luxurious types of bath products. They nourish the skin and leave it feeling silky, supple, and deliciously scented. They also make wonderful gifts. Try the recipe for Persian Lilac Bath Oil on page 193. Fill a basket with new towels, candles, a paperback book, and some scented bath products for a unique and special present.

I also like using herbs and flowers to create personal celebrations and baths for special days. Try the Zodiac Baths on page 176 or the Language of Flowers bath on page 208.

Along with choosing the right bath recipe, take the time to personalize your bath environment by using sound, color, and light. You will touch all of your senses and turn an ordinary bath into a unique experience. Place a small stereo inside your bathroom and play your favorite songs or natural sounds. Or you may prefer to hang a wind chime outside your bath window and let a gentle breeze entertain you. Color is visible light energy, and it can be used almost anywhere to create or enhance your bath-time mood. Tint your bathwater using a few drops of food coloring. Red for power, orange for independence, yellow to soothe your nerves, green (my favorite) for harmony, blue for serenity, and violet for creativity. Create a soft mood in your bath with light. The use of candlelight has become extremely popular in the bath. Scented candles are sold in almost every bath shop for just this reason—they are soothing and relaxing. You can also add a dimmer to your light switch for further control of the atmosphere. Any hardware store can provide you with one, along with easy-to-install instructions. When it comes to the bath environment, let your imagination run wild. Read poetry, place arrangements of fresh flowers or favorite artwork where you can see them, or meditate. Sometimes it's nice to enjoy a simple bath in complete silence. I fill my tub with plain hot water and then float a single flower or a slice of lemon in it to concentrate on and clear my mind.

Many of the bath recipes in this section contain dried mixtures that can be stored in clean jars with tight-fitting lids. The bath oils have long shelf lives and also can be stored in clean containers with tight-fitting lids. The bath recipes containing fresh ingredients are meant to be mixed and enjoyed the same day. The yields are enough to enjoy in one complete bath, and what remains will keep for a few days if refrigerated.

Ahh, the power of the bath . . . aside from my garden it is my most creative and enjoyable place to be!

Zodiac Baths

1 cup fresh herbs or ½ cup of dried
  herbs
Tea ball, cheesecloth, muslin bag
  (optional)

The zodiac is divided into twelve parts, each named for a constellation. We have long mused that human actions may be influenced and predicted depending upon the positions and relationships of the sun, moon, stars, and planets in the sky. Everyone has an associated sign of the zodiac determined by their birthdate and the position of the stars when they were born. Each of the twelve astrological signs also has a companion herb plant you can use to create your own personal herbal bath to celebrate your birthday. You will feel refreshed, revived, and in touch with the sky above and the cycles of nature. You can also create a very personal gift for a friend by giving them a fresh bouquet or a jar of dried zodiac herbs to enjoy in their own baths.

Herbal Astrology

Aquarius — Mullein

Pisces — Rosehip

Aries — Rosemary

Taurus — Mint

Gemini — Parsley

Cancer — Jasmine

Leo — Chamomile

Virgo — Fennel

Libra — Yarrow

Scorpio — Basil

Sagittarius — Sage

Capricorn — Comfrey

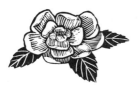

When filling your bath add the fresh or dried herbs to the bathwater either by strewing the plants directly into the water or enclosing them in a mesh container. I prefer to wrap the herbs in a piece of cheesecloth and hang it under the water faucet. This ensures a cleaner tub after bathing. When the tub is full and the herbs have steeped for a bit (about 5 minutes), bathe yourself in the warm herbal waters. You may want to carry out the astrological theme by using an afterbath splash or powder with the same scent.

Garden Note: Plant your own personal zodiac garden. In containers plant all twelve signs or just those associated with family and friends. These meaningful or personalized mini-gardens can make both special and personal presents.

Yield: 4–8 ounces, enough for one bath

These scented bath tablets dissolve in your warm bath creating a soothing and peaceful environment. Honey is one of my favorite bath additives all by itself. Combined with natural ingredients such as sea salt, clay, or dried herbs it will help restore moisture to the skin and soften your bathwater. I do not suggest doubling this recipe as the tablets must be molded while the mixture is still warm, which makes large batches hard to work with. I like to make different shapes for holiday gift-giving. I place a few tablets inside a clear cellophane bag and tie it closed with a festive bow. You will need a candy thermometer, as the correct temperature is critical in this recipe, and plastic candy molds or old ice cube trays for shaping your bath tablets.

Place the salt, clay, and dried herb leaves or flowers in a ceramic bowl or food processor bowl. Heat the honey to 300°F (hard crack). This can be done in the microwave, checking the temperature in one-minute intervals (should take 3–4 minutes total); or on the stove top,

Honey Bath Tablets

½ cup fine-grained sea salt or table salt
1 tablespoon white clay
½ tablespoon dried herb leaves or flower petals (see variations below) or use a teaspoon of the bath potpourri on page 206
½ cup pure honey

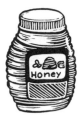

stirring the honey until the temperature reads 300°F. Pour the hot honey over the dry ingredients and stir well. You can do this with a few pulses of your food processor. Spoon the mixture into your candy molds, pressing the mixture into the molds with the back of your spoon. Let the tablets cool completely. I sometimes place them in the freezer to speed up this part of the process. Unmold your tablets onto a sheet of plastic wrap. Store them in an airtight container. To use: Place one tablet in your bath as you are filling it.

Yield: 8 ounces, 6–8 bath tablets (depending on the size of your molds)

A few variations:

You can change the scent and color of your tablets by adding different herbs, spices, and essential oils to the salt mixture. Here are a few to try:

Total Relaxation: 1 teaspoon each dried lavender flowers, marjoram leaves, and chamomile daisies

For Men Only: 1 teaspoon dried orange peel, 1 teaspoon dried bay leaves, ¼ teaspoon ground cinnamon, ½ teaspoon ground allspice

Pure Joy: 1 teaspoon dried mint, 1 teaspoon dried lavender, 2–3 drops sweet orange essential oil, 1–2 drops peppermint essential oil

Love Potion: 2 teaspoons dried rose petals, 1 small piece vanilla bean, 2–3 drops ylang-ylang oil

Myrna Loy Bath

I have always thought of Myrna Loy as the queen of Hollywood and Clark Gable as the king. Myrna was known for playing exotic women. Many of the characters she portrayed were strong, independent, and adventurous. In her 1933 hit movie The Barbarian, the star luxuriated in a petal-strewn bath. That bath scene was where I got the idea for this recipe. It is fun to try and will bring out your "inner movie star."

1 tablespoon sunflower oil
¼ cup mild liquid soap
¼ cup rosewater
2–3 drops gardenia oil or fragrance
Fresh rose petals and gardenia flowers (optional)

Stir together the oil, soap, and rosewater. Add the gardenia oil and stir well. Pour into a clean container. To use: Pour under running water as you fill the bath. For a bit of extra indulgence float fresh rose petals and gardenia flowers on top of your bathwater.

Garden Note: Gardenias are beautiful flowers with an intoxicating scent. You can wear fresh blossoms in your hair or as a corsage for a special occasion. Gardenias are good plants to grow in your bathroom since they thrive in warm, humid environments. For best results keep your plants out of direct sunlight.

Yield: 4 ounces, enough for one bath

Tub Tea

Nothing could be easier than creating a bath out of your favorite herbal tea blend. I like to envision my bathtub as one giant teapot with myself floating inside. Bathing in the soothing water and sipping a cup of my favorite blend is a wonderful and different way to enjoy afternoon tea. I simply fill a large tea ball or muslin bag with a few chosen herbs, hang it under my bath spout, and lie back! Give a friend a tea break by filling a china cup with some tub tea tied up with a gorgeous bow.

¼ cup selected combined dried herbs or ½ cup fresh herbs

Suggested blends:

- **Stimulating** — rosemary, lavender, peppermint
- **Relaxing** — chamomile, elderflower, angelica
- **Refreshing** — basil, lemon balm, mint
- **Invigorating** — raspberry leaves, bay leaves, mugwort
- **Cleansing** — sage, thyme, lemon verbena

Mix together the desired herbs. You may also use herbs individually. To use: Fill a large tea ball, muslin sack, or square of cheesecloth with the dried herbs. Hang under the bath spout as you run your bath, letting the water flow through it. Gently squeeze your tea bag or allow the tea ball to float in the bath as you bathe. After bathing discard your herbs.

Garden Note: Make your own fresh garden teas. Simply pour boiling water over some fresh leaves such as mint, chamomile, or lemon balm and let steep for a few minutes. These are always best when enjoyed in the tub.

Yield: 2–4 ounces, enough for one bath

This recipe comes from Switzerland where it is used to create refreshing, therapeutic herbal baths. It contains chlorophyll, a vital part of healthy plant life and a strong, natural deodorant. Chlorophyll is the chemical compound that absorbs light and triggers photosynthesis in all plants. You may purchase liquid chlorophyll at a natural food store or make your own (see page 182 for recipe). This bath also contains energizing herb oils such as peppermint, eucalyptus, juniper, and clove, making it a truly refreshing, exciting bath experience.

Mix together all ingredients and stir gently; do not beat or the soap will foam up. Pour the liquid into a clean container with a tight-fitting lid. To use: Pour ¼ cup into your bathwater or use in the shower as a liquid soap. Freshen and wash your skin with a thick cotton washcloth or natural body brush.

Garden Note: Growing indoor plants has been proven to improve the air quality in your home. Plants filter harmful toxins out of the air you breathe through their leaves.

Yield: 6 ounces

Swiss Green Bath

2 tablespoons liquid chlorophyll
¼ cup liquid soap
½ cup distilled water
2–3 drops essential oil of peppermint
2–3 drops essential oil of eucalyptus
2–3 drops essential oil of juniper
1 drop essential oil of clove

Make Your Own Chlorophyll

1–2 cups fresh grass clippings
1 cup vodka

*C*hlorophyll is known for its odor-absorbing properties, and for this reason it is found in many bath, body powder, and deodorant products. It also gives products a brilliant green color or tint. You may purchase liquid chlorophyll at most drug or natural food stores. It is also easy to make at home with fresh grass or alfalfa clippings. It is important that the grasses you use were not treated with any harmful chemicals—you certainly do not want pesticides or herbicides to end up in your cosmetic products.

Fill a clean jar with fresh, washed lawn clippings. Pour the vodka over the clippings. Place the lid on the jar tightly and set in a cool, dark place for 1–2 weeks. Strain off the green liquid and discard the clippings. To use: Pour ¼ cup into your bathwater. You may also use this liquid in other bath, powder, and deodorant recipes.

Yield: 8 ounces

PLANTS IN THE BATHROOM

Your bathroom provides a wonderful growing environment for many types of plants. Bright light, good ventilation, and warm, humid air make it the ideal place for houseplants. Exotic tropical plants, such as orchids and palms, that may wither and wilt in other rooms thrive in the bath. Create your own private oasis by placing one large plant or a collection of different-size plants in the bathroom's humid environment. Arrange them next to the sink, on shelves, around tubs or inside showers. Here are some of my favorite plant selections for the bath:

- Gardenia
- Orchid
- Passionflower
- Ivy
- Fern
- Creeping fig
- Coconut palm
- Spider plant
- Yucca
- Jasmine

English Lavender Bath

1 cup dried English lavender flowers
(other species may be used)
2 cups oatmeal
½ cup baking soda

There are 28 different species of lavender. English lavender is especially aromatic and one of the most widely planted varieties. All traditional herb gardens contain English lavender. This bath recipe contains lavender, as a relaxant, as well as oatmeal and baking soda, which are soothing to dry, sensitive skin. With its healing properties, this is an ideal bath for calming a bad sunburn or insect bites. Packaged inside a pretty bottle it makes a wonderful gift from the garden.

Place all the ingredients inside a food processor or blender. Grind until you have a smooth, fine powder. The powder should have the consistency of whole-grain flour. Pour into a clean, airtight container or use a resealable plastic bag. To use: Pour ½ cup into your bath as you fill the tub.

Garden Note: Prune your lavender plants immediately after they bloom to keep them compact and looking their best.

Yield: 28 ounces, enough for seven baths

Cold Comfort Bath

Scientists have yet to develop a cure for the common cold. Maybe they should take a bath? When I feel a cold coming on I immediately gather up some herbs, brew a pot of echinacea tea, and head for the bathroom. Resting in the warm, fragrant water and sipping my tea is quite comforting. After bathing, I try and stay as warm as possible—wrapping myself in a large blanket and drinking more tea. My husband also has a few tips of his own—wear only turtleneck sweaters and get lots of sleep! Use this bath when you are feeling under the weather, or make it as a thoughtful gift for a sick friend. Place a jar of it in a wicker basket filled with a box of herbal tea, vitamin C tablets, and a new book as a personal get-well wish.

2 tablespoons dried lavender flowers and leaves
2 tablespoons dried rosemary leaves
1 tablespoon dried ginger root powder
2 tablespoons dried eucalyptus leaves
Fresh eucalyptus leaves, rosemary leaves to float in bathwater (optional)

Mix together the dried herbs. Place them inside a square of natural fabric or a metal tea ball. Secure your bundle by tying the ends with a bit of string. To use: Hang the herb bag under your water tap. Fill the tub with warm (not too hot) water, letting the water flow through the herbs. Get in the bath, squeeze out your herb bag, and place it behind your neck as you bathe. You may also use it to scrub your body with a bit of soap. Note: You may also add the herbs directly to your bathwater. However, if you use this method remember that cleanup is a bit more time-consuming—something you may want to consider if you are not feeling well.

Garden Note: Purple coneflower, or echinacea, is a striking summer flower to add to your yard. It is long-stemmed and has a full, dark center with pretty purple-pink florets attached. The rhizome from the plant may be dried and used in making herbal teas. Drinking echinacea tea is believed to stimulate your immune system.

Yield: 3½ ounces

HOT BEAUTY

Heat has been used for centuries to enhance health and beauty treatments. It improves the effectiveness of baths, hair conditioning packs, and facial steams. When using heat think "warm" rather than hot. Temperatures that are too hot can be drying to your skin and hair and weaken the body. Here are some benefits you will notice after a warm bath or shower:

A glowing complexion: Warm temperatures cause your blood vessels to dilate allowing more blood to reach the skin.

Relaxed muscles: As your blood vessels dilate, more nutrients reach your tired muscles. Lactic acid produced by your muscles is also swept away by the increased bloodflow. The most relaxing bath temperature is 100°F, or just above body temperature.

Locked-in moisture: The best time to apply creams and lotions is after a warm bath or shower. Moisturizing products penetrate your skin more easily, forming a protective layer that seals in essential moisture.

Clear mind: Heat, like touch, sends positive signals to your brain, producing a relaxed, calm state of mind. This explains why we always feel better after a warm bath.

Superwoman Bath

This is the bath to take after a very full day—one in which you have leaped over small buildings, saved your co-workers, and sacrificed for family harmony. One of those rewarding yet exhausting days! One of those normal days! The scents of chamomile, rose, lavender, and hops are all soothing to women and perfect for recharging your battery before your next Super-woman adventure. This recipe can and should be doubled—for sharing!

2 tablespoons dried chamomile daisies
2 tablespoons dried rosebuds
2 tablespoons dried lavender flowers
2 tablespoons dried hops flowers

Mix together the dried flowers. Store in a clean glass jar or resealable plastic bag. To use: Place the dried flowers in the center of a square of cotton fabric. Secure the ends with a rubber band or bit of cotton string. Place in the bath as you fill your tub and allow the scented flowers to steep in the warm water.

Garden Note: Prepare a cup of this "tension taming" herbal tea. Mix together one teaspoon finely chopped or minced fresh ginger root, ¼ teaspoon finely chopped or minced fresh dandelion root, and one teaspoon pure honey in one cup boiling water. Let sit for 10–15 minutes, then strain. This tea is especially soothing when enjoyed as you soak in the bath.

Yield: 8 ounces

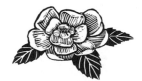

Dandelion Wine Bath

4 cups fresh dandelion flower heads
2 quarts boiling water (8 cups)
1 orange, cut into slices
1 lemon, cut into wedges
3 cups granulated or raw sugar
6 whole clove buds
2 cinnamon sticks
½ package dried yeast powder
¼ cup warm water

I recently came across this old folk recipe for dandelion wine. It made me think of a neighbor I knew while I was growing up. He made wine out of just about everything: rose hips, carrots, elderberries, and yes—dandelions. His homemade alcohols never appealed to me to drink, but it did make me think I should have used them in the bath. The fact is, people have bathed in wine for years to keep their bodies fresh and clean. Dandelion wine is well suited for this purpose, since the common yard weed is actually a cleansing tonic for tired skin. This bath recipe has a refreshing, spicy scent that will revitalize your body.

Place dandelion flowers in a glass bowl. Pour boiling water over and let sit for one week.

Strain dandelion liquid, and add orange, lemon, sugar, cloves, and cinnamon. Bring to a boil; simmer for 30 minutes. Dissolve yeast in warm water. Add yeast to saucepan and let mixture stand 2 days. Strain through coffee filters into large glass container. (I use old wine bottles.) Let stand for 3 weeks, then strain again. To use: Pour ½ cup into your bathwater and stir well.

Note: Store 3–6 months to drink as wine.

Garden Note: All parts of the dandelion plant are useful. The flowers are used to make wine and used in the bath. The leaves are rich in vitamins A and C, and when added to toner recipes help clear the skin of blemishes. The white sap is believed to help soothe and eliminate warts and corns. The roots yield a magenta-colored dye.

Yield: 64 ounces

Elizabethan Gillyflower Bath

The parent of the modern-day carnation, gillyflowers, or clove pinks as they are often called, are an aromatic, old-fashioned flower. Gillyflower was popular in Elizabethan times because of its pretty pink buds and sweet, spicy clove scent. Gillyflowers were considered a symbol of love. Engaged couples often drank from goblets with gillyflowers floating in them. Today these medieval blooms are hard to find, but the more common carnations, clove pinks, and cottage pinks can be used as substitutes. This recipe for scented bath vinegar would make a special engagement present for a young couple. Fill a basket with new bath towels, pretty soaps, fresh flowers, and a bottle of this scented bath vinegar.

1 cup fresh clove pink or carnation petals
4 cups white vinegar
6 whole clove buds

Pull the petals off the flower stems. Wash them well and pat dry. Heat vinegar to lukewarm. Place the flower petals and cloves in a large glass jar. Cover with the warm vinegar and let sit for 3 weeks. Then, strain mixture and pour into a pretty bottle with a tight-fitting lid. To use: Pour one cup of the scented vinegar into a full bath and stir well.

Garden Note: Carnations are a popular perennial flower. They can be grown from seed in a sunny location with well-drained soil.

Yield: 24 ounces, enough for four baths

Gallica Rose Bath

¼ cup rosewater

2–3 drops scented rose oil
(optional)

8 cups fresh rose petals, with a few
leaves for decoration

Gallicas are the earliest recorded roses grown. These roses are fragrant with the scent of true old rose perfume. The most famous is the Apothecary's rose (Rosa gallica officinalis), prized for its medicinal properties and bright red color. This rose is unique in that it retains its fragrance when the petals are dried. Apothecary's rose was brought to the United States by the Pilgrims and can still be found growing in many gardens today. If you are lucky enough to have this variety growing in your yard, use the fragrant petals to create this indulgent bath. If not, you may substitute another variety of fragrant rose petals. What makes this bath so luxurious is that it affects all the senses. Filling your bath with hundreds of fresh rose petals is the ultimate in pampering. It can also be very romantic when shared with someone else. Instead of sending your loved one a dozen roses, why not surprise him or her with a beautiful box full of fresh rose petals to be used in the bath?

Mix together the rosewater and rose oil. Fill the tub with warm water, adding the scented rosewater under the running water. When the tub is full, cast the fragrant rose petals into the bathwater. Slip inside the petal-filled tub and savor the moment!

Garden Note: Gallica roses are heirloom roses available through special mail-order sources. They are winter hardy and can be grown in most garden conditions. They are more adaptable to poor soils than other rose varieties.

Yield: 64 ounces of flower petals, enough for one bath

Fresh Ginger-root Bath

*F*resh gingerroot has a sweet, spicy fragrance that is also a mild stimulant. Used in the bath it promotes circulation and is perfect on a cold winter day to warm both your body and your senses. Gingerroot can easily be found at the grocery store and you can start your own plant by planting the root you buy in a pot. Keep your ginger plant in a warm, humid location, and in 8 to 12 months it should be ready to harvest. To harvest, cut off the leaf stalks and remove the fibrous roots. Cut as much as you need and replant the rest.

½ cup baking soda
2 tablespoons grated gingerroot
½ cup water

Mix together all the ingredients and pour into a clean container. To use: Pour the entire mixture into the bath as you fill the tub, stir well, and soak for 15–20 minutes. After bathing dress warmly, as this bath is super cleansing and really opens up all of your pores.

Yield: 8 ounces, enough for one bath

Harvest Moon Milk Bath

A harvest moon is defined as a full moon that occurs nearest the autumnal equinox. An equinox is when the sun crosses the equator and day and night are equal in length. In the Northern Hemisphere the first day of autumn, the equinox, is September 22 and in the Southern Hemisphere it is March 21. Celebrate this lunar phase by creating this special relaxing bath. It contains milk and almonds, both reminiscent of the large, milky moon of the equinox, and renowned for their skin softening properties.

2 cups nonfat dry milk powder
½ cup finely ground almonds or almond flour
½ cup baking soda
¼ cup bentonite clay
5–6 drops essential oil of rosemary
5–6 drops essential oil of lavender
3–4 drops essential oil of peppermint

Mix together all ingredients and pour into a clean, dry container. To use: Pour about 1 cup into the bath as you fill the tub; stir well. Soak yourself for at least 20 minutes; rinse off with a short, warm shower.

Garden Note: Some gardeners feel that the moon phases influence the activity in their gardens. Some gardening advice based on this includes: Sow corn only after a full moon; plant green beans after the change to the new moon; and never prune a tree in a full moon or it will lose its strength.

Yield: 26 ounces, enough for three baths

Scented Bath Sachets

½ cup fresh flower petals or herb
    leaves
3 tablespoons bran flour
3 pieces of natural material 6
    inches square
3 lengths of cotton string 12 inches
    long

When I suggest scattering fresh petals on your bathwater I do this for the romantic and luxurious bath effect it creates. For serious bathers interested in receiving all the therapeutic benefits of these petals, I would advise making bath sachets. They are simple to create and can be used over and over until their scent is gone. I like to use a natural muslin material for my sachets, but any scrap of pretty cotton fabric will do. Fill a large jar with several of these sachets and you will have a luxurious present for someone special.

In a bowl mix together the bran flour and flower petals or herb leaves. Place a piece of material on a flat surface and spoon one-third of the dry mixture into the center. Gather up the ends and tie them closed with the string. Place sachets in an airtight container. To use: Float one of your sachets in the bath as you fill the tub, squeezing it every now and then. You may also use it to scrub and freshen your skin as you bathe.

Yield: 6 ounces, enough for three bath sachets

Flower Power Bath

A quick and easy way to bring the benefits of flowers to your bath is to make a strong scented water using freshly picked petals. Some of my favorite flowers to use in the bath are: roses, lilac, lawn daisies, dandelions, honeysuckle, jasmine, camellia, lavender, and lily-of-the-valley. They may be used alone or in any combination you fancy. Sometimes it is fun just to gather what is blooming and use that as your bath mixture. Dried blooms may also be used for this recipe, but remember, use only half as much, as their scent is usually much stronger than fresh flowers.

½ cup fresh flower petals, removed from stem

3 cups water

Place your flower petals in a saucepan (do not use aluminum) or heat-resistant glass bowl. Pour the water over the petals. Heat the mixture until it just begins to boil—but do not boil. You may do this in either the microwave or on the stove. Remove the pan or bowl from your heat source and let sit for 20–30 minutes. Strain the liquid through a sieve, pressing down firmly on the petals to extract all of their scent and natural oils. To use: Pour this scented water into your bath as you fill the tub. If you wish, scatter some fresh flowers on the water surface and bathe among the floating petals.

Yield: 24 ounces, enough for one bath

Persian Lilac Bath Oil

The name lilac is the Persian word for "flower," and it was in that country that the plant was first discovered. In the spring I cannot wait for my lilacs to bloom. I have three beautiful bushes in my yard—white, pale lavender, and dark purple. Their heady scent is among my favorites. The fresh flowers make a luxurious bath oil that can be enjoyed year-round. You will want to make extra batches of this sweet-smelling oil to share with your friends and family.

2 cups fresh lilac flowers, removed from the main stem

1 cup castor oil

Place your flowers on a hard flat tray or cutting board. Crush each one with the back of a spoon so that it releases more of its natural scent. Pack the crushed flowers into a clean glass jar. Gently warm the castor oil on the stove or in the microwave. It should be warm to the touch but not too hot, or you will cook your flowers. Pour the warm oil over the lilacs in the jar and cover with a tight-fitting lid or cork stopper. Leave the jar in a warm place for 2 weeks. After 2 weeks, place the jar in a water bath and gently warm the contents. Remove the lid of the jar and strain out all solids from the oil. I do this by pouring the oil through a funnel lined with cheesecloth. Test your scented oil. If you desire a stronger scent, repeat the process with more fresh flowers and let sit for an additional 2 weeks. Pour your finished oil into a pretty glass bottle with a tight-fitting lid. To use: Pour a few tablespoons under your running water taps as you fill your tub.

Garden Note: When your lilacs bloom place large bouquets of the fragrant flowers throughout your home. This is an enjoyable and easy way to prune your tree and ensure blooms the following year.

Yield: 8 ounces

Winter Sunflower Soak

When added to a warm bath sunflower seeds release their rich, natural oil, leaving your skin soft and well moisturized. I also like to add to the sunflower seeds ground oatmeal, which is another well-known skin soother. This bath is a good choice during the winter months, which are marked by colder, drier weather. The change in season also lowers the humidity level outside, and your skin may appear drier, even if you have oily skin. A good 20-minute soak in this soothing bath will hydrate and soothe dry skin conditions.

¼ cup shelled, raw sunflower seeds
¼ cup oatmeal
½ teaspoon ground cinnamon
¼ teaspoon ground nutmeg
½ teaspoon vitamin E oil

In a coffee grinder or food processor, grind the sunflower seeds and oatmeal until you have a smooth powder that is the consistency of whole-grain flour. Stir in the spices and vitamin E oil and mix well. Store the mixture in an airtight container. To use: Pour the bath soak into a warm tub of water and stir well to mix. Moisturize your skin after bathing with some sunflower oil or a rich cream.

Garden Note: An old-fashioned way of cleaning garden tools for winter is to fill a bucket with sand and pour in some motor oil. Before putting your tools away, plunge them into the sand several times. The sand will scrub them, and the oil will protect them from rusting.

Yield: 4 ounces, enough for one bath

Japanese Spice Bath

1 tablespoon crushed star anise
  seeds
½ tablespoon finely chopped or
  minced fresh gingerroot
1 cup fresh pine needles
2–3 fresh chrysanthemum flowers
  (optional)

The bath is a daily ritual in Japan. The bathtub is entered after the body is thoroughly washed and rinsed. The Japanese bathe to purify themselves and soothe both the body and mind. The home bath is taken in solitude and is a time to center oneself. This is opposed to communal bathing, where conversation and the company of others is enjoyed. Natural ingredients, such as flowers, fruits, and spices, are added to the hot bathwater for medicinal, symbolic, and body-beautifying reasons. This bath contains Asian spices and fresh pine that add a pleasant scent to the water and help warm the body.

Tie the anise, ginger, and pine inside a piece of cheesecloth and hang under your tub's faucet. Fill the tub with very warm water. Float the chrysanthemum flowers on the water. Wash and scrub your body thoroughly—use a shower or faucet separate from your bathtub. Enter your tub and relax, let your mind clear—try not to think about anything in particular. When you are done soaking in the tub, rinse or shower one more time with water as cool as you can stand. Towel dry, and apply a light bath oil to lock in your skin's moisture.

Garden Note: Japanese-style gardens are so simple in design yet elegant. They have privacy, serenity, and an air of mystery about them. If you are lucky enough to live near one I would definitely suggest a visit. If you like, you can study them and plant a garden of your own that you can enjoy every day.

Yield: 8 ounces, enough for one bath

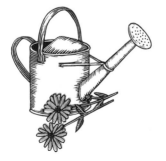

Oh, What a Beautiful Mornin'! Shower Gel

One of my favorite feel-good songs of all time is Rodgers and Hammerstein's 1943 hit from the Broadway musical Oklahoma! *What better way to start your day than with an invigorating shower and a rousing chorus of "Oh, What a Beautiful Mornin'!" This recipe contains fresh marjoram and eucalyptus, both of which are naturally antiseptic and refreshing to your skin. You may also use this as a bath enhancer.*

Place the eucalyptus, marjoram, and cinnamon stick in a glass bowl. Pour the boiling water over them and allow the mixture to steep for several hours, until cool. Strain off the liquid and mix with the liquid soap and glycerine. Pour the soap solution into a clean, plastic container with a pour spout. To use: Apply as you would any liquid soap or shower gel, or pour into the bath under running water.

2 tablespoons fresh marjoram
1 cup fresh eucalyptus leaves
1 small cinnamon stick
1 cup boiling water
½ cup liquid soap
1 tablespoon glycerine

Garden Note: Make a rich compost tea for your garden to enjoy. Wrap a shovelful of compost with several layers of cheesecloth, tie the ends closed with string, and place the "tea bag" in a pail of water to steep overnight. Use this solution to give stressed plants a boost of nutrients or as a general fertilizer. You can also spread the used compost around your garden after you are done with it.

Yield: 12 ounces

Xena, Warrior Princess Bath

½ cup crushed almonds or almond
  flour
1 cup baking soda
1 cup fresh pine needles
2 tablespoons juniper berries
6 bay leaves

A recent television phenomenon is the popularity of a fictitious warrior princess named Xena. Out of the golden age of mythology and legends, she is truly a heroine for all ages. Surrounded by evil enemies, barbaric tribes, and slave traders, Xena's mission is to help people free themselves from tyranny and injustice. She kicks, punches, and howls her way to victory. If ever there was a woman who needed a good, hot bath after facing the evil of the world it is Xena. This recipe is for an amazing, aromatic bath guaranteed to soothe tired, overworked muscles.

Place all the ingredients in a blender or food processor and grind until you have a coarse, fragrant mixture. Spoon approximately ½ cup of this mixture into a muslin tea bag or onto the center of a square of cheesecloth and tie the ends with a bit of cotton string. Store bags in an airtight container. To use: Fill your tub with warm water and allow the bath bag to float in the water, giving it a gentle squeeze every now and then. Use this same bag to scrub the body all over.

Yield: 16 ounces, 3–4 bath bags

Pauline's Silk Milk Bath

2 cups dried nonfat milk powder
¼ cup slippery elm powder
1 tablespoon honey
2 cups boiling water
4–5 drops fine perfume or selected
  essential oils (optional)

*T*he Bonaparte family was a very close and powerful Corsican clan. Joseph was king of Naples and Spain, Napoleon a famous French general, Lucien the prince of Canino, and Louis the king of Holland. Their sister, Pauline, married Prince Borghese and, like her brothers, was also quite ambitious. This made for a very tumultuous marriage with Pauline often going off on her own. She was also known to be an incredible beauty and loved using cosmetics and heavy perfumes. Bathing in milk was one of her favorite beauty indulgences. This recipe calls for dried milk, slippery elm powder, and pure honey and is meant to replicate the baths that I believe made Pauline's skin "feel of fine silk."

Combine the dried milk, elm powder, and honey in a glass pitcher or bowl. Add the boiling water and stir well until all the powders are dissolved. To use: Draw a warm bath and pour the entire milk mixture into the water; stir well. Soak in the tub for at least 20 minutes. Rinse the milk off your skin with cool water and pat yourself dry. Moisturize your body with a rich oil.

Garden Note: Slippery elm powder is made from the dried inner bark of the slippery elm tree (*Ulmus rubra*). It is available at many grocery and natural food stores.

Yield: 16 ounces, enough for one bath

Mariann's Eucalyptus Bath

My sister, Mariann, lives in California. In her backyard she has a fragrant eucalyptus tree. Whenever she prunes her tree, she shares her clippings with my mother and me. When this happens, I instantly begin preserving them by cooking up lotions, oils, and this bath recipe. Any remaining stems I use in floral arrangements and potpourri blends to give my house a fresh, clean scent. This recipe is quick and easy to make. It is extremely refreshing, and perfect for a morning bath or to cool off on a hot day.

2 cups fresh eucalyptus leaves, well rinsed
4 cups water
½ teaspoon castor oil

Gently tear or bruise your eucalyptus leaves to release their fragrant natural oils. Place the leaves in a medium-size saucepan. Cover them with water, and over medium heat gently warm them for 20 minutes. Do not boil. Allow the mixture to cool completely and then stir in the castor oil. This acts as a scent fixative. Pour the scented water into a clean container. To use: Pour about a cup of this bath water into a tub of warm water. Note: The cooler your bath temperature the more energizing your bath will be.

Garden Note: Hang a sprig of fresh eucalyptus inside your bath or shower to freshen the air as you bathe. The heat and humidity in the air will release its uplifting scent.

Yield: 32 ounces, enough for four baths

Thyme Out

½ cup fresh thyme leaves and
   flowers
2 cups cold water
5–6 drops essential oil of thyme
   (optional)

Sometimes we all need a time out, or rather a thyme out. When you want to collect your thoughts and refresh your body reach for your pot of thyme and head for the bathroom. Thyme has been used for centuries as a cleansing, invigorating bath. The name thyme *comes from the Greek word for courage,* thymus, *and is appropriate for such an exhilarating herb. Roman soldiers bathed in thyme water to give themselves power and strength.*

Gently tear or bruise the thyme leaves to release their fragrant natural oils. Place the leaves in a medium-size saucepan. Cover with water and gently warm for 20 minutes; do not boil. Allow the mixture to cool completely and then add the essential oil, if you desire a stronger scent. Pour the scented water into a clean container. To use: Pour into your bath and stir well.

Garden Note: Plant creeping thyme between stepping-stones or as a ground cover. When walked on, the leaves release an aromatic, light fragrance with faint notes of citrus.

Yield: 16 ounces, enough for one bath

Extreme Soak

E xtreme *seems to be the new buzzword. We now live in a world full of extreme drinks, clothes, and sports — so why not an extreme bath as well? These soothing bath salts contain bay and marjoram, both known for stimulating circulation and comforting sore muscles. They make an outrageous soak for an ultra-tired body. I grind the dried leaves to a fine powder, making them extremely aromatic and effective.*

¼ cup dried bay leaves
¼ cup dried marjoram leaves
1 cup baking soda
2 cups fine sea salt

Grind the dried herbs in a coffee grinder or food processor until you have a fine, green powder. In a large bowl mix together all ingredients and stir well. Pour into an airtight container. To use: Pour ½ cup of this bath mixture into the bath. Store any remaining bath in a dry, airtight container.

Garden Note: When growing marjoram cut off the blossoms and keep the plant trimmed to prevent the stems from growing too woody. Marjoram is an attractive indoor plant if given enough sun.

Yield: 28 ounces, enough for seven baths

Bath Salts

B ath *salts are some of my easiest recipes to make and some of my most popular. They are wonderful and welcome presents for just about everyone and you can tailor their scents and colors for each recipient. Besides soothing tired bodies and softening skin, these salts are also easier on the bathtub than other products. They are ideal bath additives because they actually help keep your tub clean. They are so soluble in water that they do not leave any residues behind. Because of this, bath salts are often recommended by whirlpool manufacturers. They do not clog the pipes as other bath products can. Bath salts also soften hard water. Soap does not clean well in hard water, nor does it lather well. In soft water, however, it creates lots of bubbles and is more effective at cleaning your skin. Bath salts help keep your water temperature warmer longer, too. Natural salts are easily found at the grocery store.*

Following are a few of my favorite methods for making bath salts. Start with a basic salt mix of one cup Epsom salts and one cup rock salt (you can use kosher salt, sea salt, or rock table salt).

Colored salts: You can successfully color your salts with regular food coloring or natural vegetable dyes, such as beet juice. For more exotic colors check out cake decorating shops that sell paste-style food dyes. Place your salts in a large glass bowl or resealable plastic bag. Add a few drops of color and stir well, or massage the bag until the color is well mixed. If you desire a darker shade add more color. If your color is too dark, add more salt. Be careful when making very dark salts; until they are diluted in your bathwater they may stain light-colored towels and clothing. Once added to your bath they will not stain your skin or tub. My daughters like to make rainbow salts by creating salts in several different colors and then layering them like a rainbow inside a pretty jar.

Scented salts: Fragrance can be added to your natural salts as well as color. The method is the same as in adding color. Simply stir or massage scented oils into your salt mixture. Choose oil-based scents and essential oils; these tend to be stronger and longer lasting. You only need a few drops to scent a batch of salts. You may also combine scented oils to create your own special blends. For example: Create bathtime tranquillity with a blend of sweet orange oil, vanilla oil, and carnation oil.

Foaming salts: Any bath salt recipe can be made to foam in the tub by adding mild liquid soap to your mixture. To do this mix your color and/or scent into the liquid soap before stirring it into the salt mixture. I use ¼ cup liquid soap for every 2 cups of salt. Mix the soap with your salt and then spread the mixture on a clean cookie sheet and allow it to air-dry completely. To speed up this process, you may place the salts in a low temperature oven or food dehydrator. When your salts are completely dry, pour them into an airtight container.

Herbal salts: Adding dried herbs and flower petals to your basic mix gives your salts a different look as well as a wonderfully natural feel. You will also receive many of the benefits that adding herbs to your bath can provide. I like to use 1–2 tablespoons of a dried herb or combination of herbs to every 2 cups of the basic salt mixture. It is important that you use dried ingredients rather than fresh in making these salts. Fresh leaves and petals wilt when they come in contact with the salt, releasing unwanted moisture into your mixture.

To use any of these bath salts: Add about ½ cup of bath salts to your tub under the running water. Store your salts in dry, airtight containers.

Yield: 16 ounces, enough for four baths

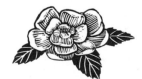

Bathing Outdoors

*R*oll the roof off your bathroom and enjoy complete cleansing freedom. If you have never taken a shower or bath outdoors, you don't know what you are missing! It is the ultimate way to enjoy nature, with the sky overhead, plants and trees around you, and the sounds of nature as your stereo system. All of your senses will become awakened and refreshed.

The construction of your outdoor bathroom can be as simple as hanging a solar shower over a tree branch or as complex as installing standard plumbing hardware in your yard. You pick the spot—the back of your garden shed, under a grape arbor, against an ivy-covered wall. Wherever you can find access to water, good drainage, and a bit of privacy is perfect for your natural shower spot. You may want to plant a hedge, build a fence, or construct a vine-covered trellis to provide cover around your chosen place. Bathing outdoors also has its functional points. It is a great way to clean up after gardening or at the end of a day at the beach, leaving mud and sand outdoors where it belongs.

Drainage is essential for your bathing spot. All of that wash water has to go somewhere. You may want to dig a large hole and fill it with gravel. Place a wooden slatted bath mat over this spot to stand on while bathing.

Privacy is important and also a matter of personal choice. Your location may be private enough, or you can construct a number of "walls" for your bathing peace of mind. My friend Leslie made a wonderfully simple enclosure by her pool using PVC pipe and shower curtains. She created a frame with PVC pipes and standard pipe joints (check your local hardware store) and used three standard shower curtains and rings to enclose her spot. To stabilize the legs of her enclosure she set them in heavy clay pots filled with sand and gravel.

Bathtubs are also wonderful when moved outdoors. Today many houses have outdoor hot tubs, pools, and spas for this reason. These are a bit different than an actual tub, since people rarely wash with soap and water in them. But these private watering holes are a great way to unwind at the end of the day with a good soaking. If you do not want to install a traditional tub, try using a child's inflatable swimming pool outdoors in your yard or patio. If you fill it in the morning and let the sun warm the water all day it should be quite enjoyable in the late afternoon.

So, whether you strip off all your clothes and run through the sprinklers, wash off the mud after a day in the garden, or fill an old bath full of flowers under a starry sky, bathing outdoors is one of life's simple pleasures that should be experienced.

Scented Bath Pillow

Create a fragrant rest for your head to use while bathing. All you need is a cotton towel, some dried herbs, and a couple of suction cups from your local hardware store. This pillow also makes a nice present for a special friend, especially if included with a jar of scented bath salts (see page 201). You will need a standard size cotton bath towel, 24 x 44 inches, or a piece of cotton terry cloth material, 2 plastic suction cups from the hardware store, 2 pieces of cotton ribbon or cord, each 18 inches in length, and a needle and thread.

1 cup dried herb mixture (lavender, rose petals, rosemary)

Place the bath towel on a flat work surface. Fold the towel lengthwise. Sprinkle the towel with the dried herbs. Starting at one end, roll up the towel. Tie a length of ribbon or cord around each end to keep it rolled up and the herbs in place. Stitch or glue the suction cups to the ribbons on the back of the pillow. To use: Secure to the back of your tub, under your head. The pillow may be undone by untying the ribbons. This allows you to wash the towel and replace the herbs when their scent has disappeared.

Yield: 1 pillow

THE LANGUAGE OF FLOWERS

You can create unique and special bath bouquets and bath potpourri by practicing the Victorian art of using flowers to express your feelings. This is a special and individual way to communicate with a friend or loved one. Listed below is a sampling of the more than 700 flowers and herbs and the meaning that was attached to them in the early 1900s. You may choose one simple flower to convey your thoughts, such as a single rose for love, or a whole floral response containing daisies, I share your sentiments; chervil, sincerity; and red tulips, a declaration of love.

Allspice — Compassion

Aloe — Affection

Amaranth — Unfading love

Alyssum — Worth beyond beauty

Amaryllis — Pride

Angelica — Inspiration

Apple blossoms — Temptation

Birch leaves — Meekness

Blue salvia — I think of you

Borage flowers — Bluntness

Cabbage — Profit

Cactus — Warmth

Chamomile — Energy in adversity

Cedar — Strength

Daffodil — Regard

Dahlia — Good taste

Elm leaves — Patriotism

Fennel — Worthy of all praise

Fern — Sincerity

Flowering almond — Hope

Forget-me-nots — True love

Grass — Submission

Holly — Foresight

Hollyhock — Productivity

Hyacinth — Sport, game, play

Ice plant — Your looks "freeze" me

Ivy — Friendship

Lemon — Zest

Mint — Virtue

Oak leaves — Bravery

Palm fronds — Victory

Petunia — Never despair

Stock — Lasting beauty

Thyme — Activity

Water lily — Purity of heart

Zinnia — Thoughts of absent friends

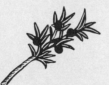

THE ULTIMATE GARDEN BATH

To create a whimsical garden feature in your garden, plant an herb garden inside an old bathtub. Shop secondhand shops, flea markets, and garage sales for an old tub. Place the tub in the center of your garden and fill it with planting soil. Place your favorite herb plants, such as lavender, chamomile, and mint, inside. Water it well and in a few months it will be overflowing with herbs and flowers—the ultimate garden bath!

Body Care Products and Treatments

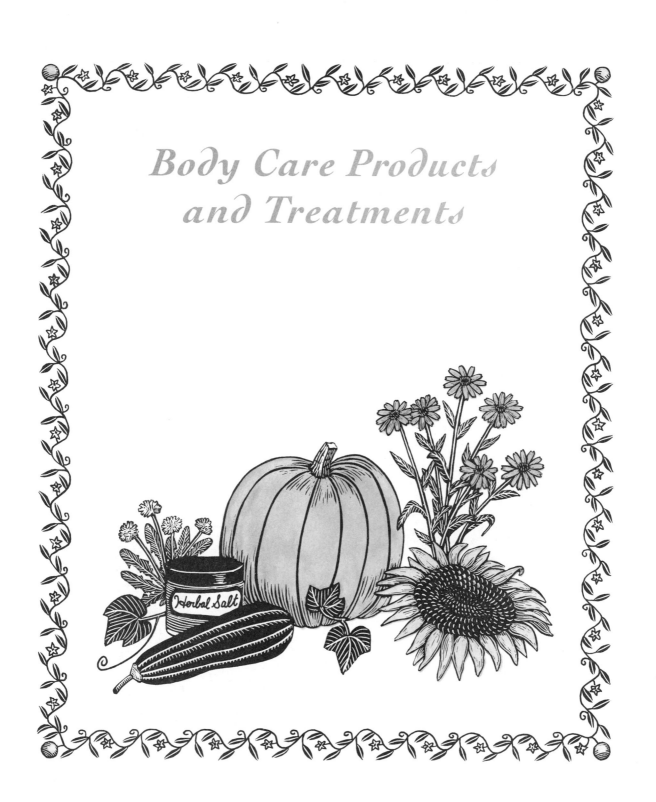

*C*ultivate one's own garden" is a popular expression. To me it means: Take care of yourself first. This may seem a bit selfish, but I like to think of it this way—the better you feel the better you will make others feel. I know from personal experience that I am at my best and most effective when I have taken time out for myself. This can be something as basic as eating breakfast or as indulgent as a Botanical Body Wrap (see page 216). My point is, however you choose to do it, you should take care of yourself first! Body care products and treatments are an ideal way to do this. Some I have included are practical and others are pure luxury. Use a combination of both; experiment and expand your beauty range.

Our skin is the largest organ of the body. It protects the body from the environment, enhances our sense of touch, and regulates our body's temperature. Taking time to care for it is very important. To do so is a basic three-step routine. The latest tools, gadgets, and decorative touches are fun to try in the garden, but if your plants do not get the basics such as water, food, and sunshine they will not grow. The same principles are true with skin care. If your skin does not get proper regular attention, it will not look its best, regardless of the cosmetics or latest advanced beauty treatments you try. I always say there are three main areas in maintaining healthy skin: (1) keeping it clean; (2) keeping it full of moisture; and (3) keeping it protected from the sun. The products and treatments you choose to address these three areas are a matter of personal preference. You can use a simple soap for cleansing and natural oils or expensive commercial beauty formulas for moisture. Whichever you choose, the end results are basically the same. Correct skin care is really more about common sense than spending money on the latest cleanser, cream, or lotion. In this section you will find simple yet effective recipes for keeping your skin clean, moist, and radiant. I have also included some at-home spa treatments for that extra indulgence we can all use.

One of my favorite treatments is the full-body scrub. Full-body scrubs not only feel great but also help rid your skin of surface impurities and dead skin cells. This enables your skin to retain more moisture. Use the recipe for the Herbal Salt Rub on page 218 and experience a spa-style treatment in the privacy of your own home. Your skin will feel revitalized and have a healthy sheen. On the more practical side, you'll see I've included several natural deodorant products that can be made from plants. Ancient Egyptians used to walk around with henna leaves under their arms to ward off "evil" smells. I would not necessarily recommend this, but I would advise the use of sweet-smelling botanicals such as lovage, witch hazel, and fresh citrus peels to keep yourself feeling fresh all day naturally.

Another important and necessary product I have included is a make-at-home sunscreen, but I don't recommend this for fair-skinned readers or children as it doesn't provide enough sun protection. It is difficult to create a totally natural product with a sun protection factor (SPF) higher than 8. The sun is important to all growing things and sunlight is necessary for good health, but care should be taken when you are outside. The threat of skin cancer and sun damage is real. Gone are the days of worshipping the sun without proper protection. Overexposure to the sun can also break down collagen, the protein substance that gives the skin elasticity, making wrinkles and lines more apparent. This is why, when gardening or enjoying the outdoors, it is so important to protect any exposed skin. Avoid being outside in direct sunlight during the middle of the day. This is when the rays of the sun are strongest. A good way to test this is to check your shadow—if it is larger than you are, the sun is not directly overhead and you are safe. If not, you want to be sure you have the right supplies or stay out of the sun until later in the day. A good pair of sunglasses and a wide-brimmed hat are two of your best beauty tools. They will slow down wrinkling around the eyes and protect your face from the sun's harmful rays.

From the summer's heat to the winter's cold and every day in between, remember that your skin longs to be moist. In this section there are several rich moisturizing body lotions that you can use all over after bathing, or whenever your skin needs more moisture. Remember, dry skin is not caused by loss of skin oils but by the loss of water. Body oils and lotions create a protective barrier on the skin surface, locking in moisture and slowing down its evaporation. One of the most effective times to apply body lotions is after bathing. Just out of the tub or shower, your skin is full of water and the heat from the bath helps the cream penetrate deeply into every pore. Make moisturizing a habit after every long soak.

The garden is a great place to throw a garden party (see page 214) and share your herbs and flowers with a few special friends. You may want to have a beauty workshop party where you and your friends make some of the recipes from this book together.

Whether you make them with friends or on your own, store your body creams and lotions in clean containers in a cool, dark location. Many of the full-body treatment recipes make enough for one to two applications. Always store leftover products that contain fresh ingredients in the refrigerator to extend their shelf life.

Schedule some time for yourself and whip up some potions to pamper your skin from head to toe. Your body can use some special attention, and nature provides the most healing ingredients. Brush, buff, scrub, soothe, and energize yourself!

GARDEN PARTY BEAUTY

Plan a wonderful feel-good afternoon outside for you and your friends. Call up a few friends, brew a pot of herbal tea, and share your garden with them. Move your stereo system outdoors to play your favorite recorded music and set the party mood. Cover a picnic table with a pretty linen cloth and set out all the necessary tools for manicures, pedicures, and facial masks. Have some garden and beauty books and magazines on hand for your guests to read as they pamper themselves. Together, you can create and put to immediate use a few of the recipes from this book. Herbal bath products, scented perfumes, and facial toners are all easy and fun to make. You may also want to send home clippings from some of your favorite herbs and flowers for your friends to plant in their own gardens.

Dry Brushing

Dry brushing is a popular spa treatment that you can easily do yourself at home before bathing. This treatment opens up clogged pores by removing dead skin cells and surface debris. The boost it gives your skin's circulation is also believed to eliminate cellulite.

Dry brushing is simple and takes about 5 to 10 minutes. You should try it head to toe before bathing. You will want to start out gently, and, once your skin is used to this type of treatment, work your way up to more vigorous brushing. Note: Never use dry brushing on your face, and women should avoid the breast area.

To try this treatment you will need a soft, natural fiber body brush the size of your palm. Dry brushing is done on dry skin—do not use lotions, oils, or water on your skin or the brush. Just begin brushing your hands first, followed by the arms, neck, chest, stomach, and back. Brush in smooth, flowing strokes and do not apply too much pressure. This treatment should feel pleasurable, not painful. Now go on to each leg, starting at the foot. When you are finished you will feel invigorated and your skin will be glowing.

Following dry brushing you should shower or bathe as you usually do, washing away all the dead skin cells you just exfoliated from your body. Your skin will feel incredibly clean and soft. You should also feel healthier. Many people believe dry brushing removes toxins from their entire system. When you step from the bath do not rub your skin dry, but pat it with a warm fluffy towel and apply a light skin oil or moisturizer.

Keep your dry brush clean by washing it in a mild soap once a week and allowing it to air-dry completely.

Botanical Body Wrap

1 cup fresh mint leaves
1 cup fresh lavender flowers
1 cup fresh sage leaves
½ cup dried fennel seeds

Body wraps are hot, and I am not talking about their temperature. This spa-style treatment, which was once only found in the most exclusive European resorts, has become extremely popular with modern women and men. It is now practiced in almost every major beauty salon in the world. Even in my small Oregon town, I can book a "wrap" session. The procedure involves dry brushing or scrubbing the body, deeply moisturizing it with oil, and then encasing it in herb-soaked towels to tone and moisturize the skin. The purpose of all this is to deep-cleanse and relax your whole body. This recipe is my garden version of this popular treatment. It works best if you have a partner to help wrap you up. You will need a plastic drop cloth from the hardware store or a plastic shower curtain, and a large cotton bed sheet for this treatment.

Place the plastic shower curtain on top of your bed or a carpeted spot on the floor where you can rest during your wrap. Place the fresh herbs inside a large ceramic bowl or plastic bucket. Fill this container with very hot tap water and let sit for 5 minutes. Soak your sheet in this solution. Now prepare your body by gently dry brushing your skin all over (see page 215 for instructions.) Massage a favorite scented oil into your skin or simply use light sesame oil. Wring out the hot wet sheet and wrap it snugly around your body. Lie down on the plastic drop cloth and have your partner help you wrap yourself in it. Cover yourself with blankets and lie quietly for no more than 10 minutes. Try not to talk or be distracted. Just enjoy the wonderful sense of relaxation this treatment provides! After 10 minutes is up, slowly unwrap yourself and get up. You should feel fresh and revitalized!

Garden Note: I just read in one of my beauty magazines that we should all practice more "ecotherapy." This big word simply means spending more time in natural settings. What better place to treat your mind and body than in your garden? I know a few hours among the plants makes me as relaxed and centered as any of the more complicated and costly options available today. Try it for yourself and see!

Yield: 1 full body wrap

Dandelion Age Spot Oil

The name dandelion *comes from the French* dent de lion, *or "lion's tooth," because the plant leaves are so deeply jagged. Many people consider dandelions an annoying weed because they overtake lawns and gardens, but they are actually very useful beauty-wise. The yellow flowers make a wonderful bath and hair rinse. The green leaves are rich in vitamins A and C. Many people add them to their salads. In this recipe they are used to naturally fade away stubborn freckles and brown age spots.*

¼ cup fresh, chopped dandelion
   leaves
2 tablespoons castor oil
2 tablespoons sunflower oil

Make sure the dandelion leaves are clean and dry; pat with a clean towel to remove excess moisture. Place the leaves and oils in a heat-resistant container and gently warm. Do not boil. Let the mixture sit for at least 3 hours. Strain out all the leaves and pour into a clean bottle with a tight-fitting cork or lid. To use: Rub a small amount of the oil into your skin daily. It may take several weeks, but you will soon see your freckles and age spots begin to fade.

Garden Note: As we all know, dandelions are easy to grow. Collect wild seeds—those fluffy puffballs children love to blow—and plant them in a corner of your garden. They will grow in almost every soil type.

Yield: 2 ounces

Herbal Salt Rub

2 cups sea salt or kosher salt

½ cup sweet almond oil

¼ cup macadamia nut oil (if this is hard to find, use light olive oil)

¼ cup light sesame oil

1 teaspoon vitamin E oil

1 tablespoon dried rosemary, spearmint, and lavender combined

1–2 drops essential oil for scent (optional)

A favorite spa offering around the world is a salt rub. This full-body treatment combines exfoliation, moisturization, and light massage for the ultimate skin pampering experience. Coarse salt is mixed together with natural oils and dried herbs, then rubbed all over the body to make your skin feel like velvet. The salt removes dead skin cells and other surface impurities as the oils simultaneously lubricate and soothe the skin. The big secret is that because this treatment is so simple, a spa-quality salt rub can easily be done in the privacy of your own home. This recipe makes a luxurious gift for a friend who could use a feel-good glow all over his/her body—and who couldn't?

Mix together the salt, oils, and herbs, and stir well to form a thick paste. Pour into a clean jar with a tight-fitting lid. To use: While standing in the tub or shower, take a handful of the paste and gently massage it into your skin, starting with your feet (be careful, as the oil will make them very slippery). Massage the paste all over your body. When you have finished this and your body is covered, rinse with warm water and pat your skin dry. Do not use soap or other cleansers, as this will remove the oil and spoil the treatment's lovely moisturizing effect. Save any leftover rub in a clean container. It will keep for 1–2 months and does not need refrigeration.

Yield: 16 ounces

Southwest Scrub

Blue cornmeal is an ancient food that also makes a rejuvenating full-body treatment. The Hopi Indians of New Mexico have used blue cornmeal for years to improve vitality and make their skin look more youthful. Mixing it with dried herbs, ground oatmeal, and a mild soap enhances this age-old cleanser. If you cannot find blue cornmeal at your market, you may substitute white or yellow cornmeal for a differently colored but just as effective scrub.

½ cup ground blue cornmeal
½ cup grated castile soap (or other mild bar soap)
¼ cup oatmeal
1 teaspoon dried calendula flower petals
½ teaspoon dried rosemary leaves
1 teaspoon dried lavender flowers

Place the cornmeal and grated soap in a large bowl. Using a spice or coffee grinder, finely grind the oatmeal and dried herbs. Add this mixture to the cornmeal mixture and stir well. Pour into a clean, airtight container. To use: Apply as you would any cleanser, and massage all over your body. Rinse well and then moisturize your skin with a natural oil or rich body lotion. If you have very sensitive skin avoid using this cleanser on your face.

Yield: 12 ounces

Geranium Petal Body Scrub

This sweet-scented body scrub is perfect for freshening and moisturizing the skin. Body scrubs are helpful because they stimulate circulation. A gentle rubdown can counteract stress, help rid the body of excess fluid, and really energize your whole system. This is a good all-over treatment to use during your morning shower. I like to use raw sugar for its coarse texture and subtle molasses scent. People with oily skin should reduce the amount of walnut oil called for in this recipe—or leave it out completely.

1 cup raw sugar
12 dried geranium flower heads
¼ cup walnut oil
½ teaspoon vitamin E oil
1–2 drops essential oil of geranium

Mix together all the ingredients in a large glass or ceramic bowl. Spoon into a clean jar with a tight-fitting lid. To use: Massage a tablespoon or two all over your body to gently exfoliate and moisturize your skin. Store any remaining scrub in a cool, dry location. You may need to stir the product between uses.

Yield: 10 ounces, enough for 4–5 full-body treatments

Jack-o'-Lantern Body Mask

3–4 cups fresh pumpkin flesh with seeds

*M*y daughters love to grow pumpkins for Halloween. They delight in imagining the funny, scary "jack-o'-lanterns" they will make. I tend to appreciate pumpkins as beneficial beauty ingredients. So, every October as we hollow out our large, orange gourds, I save the insides for making this skin-beautifying body mask. Pumpkin contains fruit acid enzymes that work like alpha hydroxy acid. The real plus is that these enzymes remove dead skin cells with less irritation than commercial products. The lovely orange pulp also has anti-inflammatory properties, making it naturally soothing. This treatment is well suited for all skin types, especially sensitive ones.

In a food processor, process the pumpkin flesh for 1–2 minutes until you have a smooth, grainy puree. To use: Standing in the tub or on an old bath towel, massage the pumpkin mixture into your skin starting at your feet and working your way up. This mask is mild enough to be used on your face. Let the mask rest on your skin for 5 minutes. Then, rinse your skin in a warm bath or shower and pat dry. You may keep any leftover mask in the refrigerator or frozen for future use.

Garden Note: For Halloween pumpkins the key is to plant early. Many of my friends start their plants in May for an October harvest.

Yield: 16 ounces, enough for two body masks

It is important to eat plenty of fresh fruits and vegetables, which help to produce healthy skin and hair from the inside out. But today fresh "green" ingredients are also something to put on your body. These ingredients come from the vegetable patch and smell a bit like a freshly tossed salad as they add moisture to your skin, making it feel soft and smooth.

Combine all the fresh vegetables in a steamer or micro-wave-safe container. Steam until they are soft and tender and can easily be pierced with a fork. Let the vegetables cool completely and save ½ cup of their cooking water as the vegetable water. Place the cooked vegetables and water in a blender or food processor and process until smooth. Using a fork or whisk, stir in the natural clay (see page 107 for more about clays). When you finish mixing you should have a smooth, pale-green, creamy mixture. To use: Spread the mask all over your body using your fingers or a small pastry brush. Let the mixture sit on your skin for 10–15 minutes. Wrap an old towel around yourself and lie down if you like. Rinse off the body mask in a warm shower and use a rich moisturizer afterward.

Garden Note: Use your old panty hose to protect your ripening squash so that birds and other garden pests do not nibble on them. Simply pull a leg over each squash and tie them off at each end. As your squash grows the stretchy fabric will expand with it.

Yield: 10 ounces, enough for one treatment

Green Body Mask

1 cup sliced fresh carrot root
2 cups fresh spinach leaves
½ cup sliced mushrooms
1 cup fresh, sliced zucchini squash
½ cup vegetable water (see instructions below) or fresh water
½ cup French green clay or white China clay

Poison Ivy

Remember the old camp rhyme, "Leaflets of three, let it be"? Poison ivy and poison oak are both vigorously growing vines with three-leaf clusters. Learn to identify them and keep your distance. These plants contain an oil that can cause an itchy red rash with small blisters when it comes into contact with your skin. If you have run into one of these plants, the faster you can wash the affected area the better your chances are of preventing a bad rash. Wash the affected spot with plenty of soap and water that is as hot as you can stand. Be sure to clean carefully under your fingernails.

Follow up your initial washing with soap and water showers every 3 or 4 hours for the next 24 hours. Also, wash your clothing—throw everything from shoes (if you can) to underwear in the washing machine and use a strong laundry detergent to flush out those plant oils, or they'll get you again.

If you do break out, soothe the rash with a solution of equal parts milk and water or salt water (¼ cup salt to one cup water). Soak strips of cotton cloth in either of these solutions and lay them on your skin. Wash your skin often and gently, making sure not to rub the affected areas, which could spread your rash.

If the itchiness is more than you can stand, run a warm bath and add two cups oatmeal or baking soda to the bathwater. Soak in the bath. After bathing, pat your skin dry and let the powdery residue from the oatmeal or soda remain. It will help keep the itching down.

Try, try, try not to scratch. This can spread the rash and even lead to infection. If the outbreak does not improve with these home treatments check with your physician. He or she may be able to prescribe topical or oral medications that will reduce your discomfort while the rash runs its course.

Summer solstice is the longest day of the year. The sun begins to move lower in the sky and the days begin to get shorter. In the Northern Hemisphere this occurs on June 21 and in the Southern Hemisphere on December 21. To celebrate this day of extra light and sunshine mix up a batch of this rich cream made from fresh flowers and herbs from your garden. Use it on your skin until winter solstice, when the days will begin to increase once again.

Place the flowers, leaves, and borax in a ceramic or glass dish. Pour the boiling water over them and allow the mixture to cool completely. Strain the mixture, saving the liquid. Combine the oils and beeswax, and heat gently until the beeswax is melted. You may do this using a double boiler over medium heat or in the heat-resistant container in a microwave. Heat the herbal liquid gently over medium heat until it just begins to boil. Remove from heat, and pour the hot liquid into a blender or food processor. Start stirring and slowly add the oil mixture, pouring it in a thin, even stream. Blend until you have a smooth cream. Let the cream cool completely, stirring occasionally. Spoon into a clean container with a tight-fitting lid. To use: Massage into your skin.

Yield: 8 ounces

Summer Solstice Cream

½ cup boiling water
1 tablespoon fresh lavender flowers
1 tablespoon fresh parsley leaves
½ teaspoon fresh chamomile flowers
⅛ teaspoon borax powder
½ cup sunflower oil
1 teaspoon grapeseed oil
2 tablespoons grated beeswax

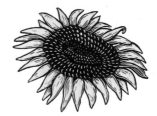

Love-in-a-Mist Lotion

⅛ teaspoon borax powder
¼ cup distilled water
1 tablespoon love-in-a-mist
    (nigella) seeds, crushed
¼ cup sweet almond oil
¼ cup grapeseed oil
1 tablespoon grated beeswax

Ancient Egyptian women ate nigella seeds to beautify and firm their breasts. Roman women massaged a strong tea made from the seeds onto their torsos and also created a powder made from the ground seeds to rub into their breasts at night "to restore feminine beauty and freshness." Also known as Roman coriander, this annual has pale blue flowers that appear amid feathery foliage, thus the nickname love-in-a-mist. The small black seeds have a spicy aroma like nutmeg. Traditionally this potion was intended for the upper torso, but I have found it makes a wonderful full-body moisturizer.

Combine the borax and water and heat until mixture starts to boil. Then pour it over the love-in-a-mist seeds and let steep for 15–20 minutes until cool. In another container mix together the oils and beeswax and heat until the beeswax is melted. Strain the water solution and heat to roughly the same temperature as the oil mixture. Pour the oil mixture into a blender and start stirring; slowly add the water solution and then mix on High until a thick lotion is formed. Pour the lotion into a cool container and allow it to cool completely. To use: Massage into your skin as you would any rich moisturizer or cream.

Garden Note: Nigella seeds can be ordered from a number of seed sources and are available at many garden centers. Pale blue is the most common flower color, but other varieties will produce shades such as white, rose, and yellow. Nigellas are annuals that bloom from late spring through summer.

Yield: 8 ounces

Natural Deodorants

Perspiration is a normal, healthy part of our body's cooling system. It helps regulate body temperature and releases salts and toxic substances from the body. Fresh perspiration is basically odorless, but when left to mix with bacteria on our skin's surface it can cause a not-so-pleasant odor. So, to stay smelling fresh it is important to keep your skin clean, especially after a strenuous task or exercising, when your body tends to perspire more. The use of a deodorant product is also helpful in combating body odor.

There are two main types of products that can be used — antiperspirants and deodorants. An antiperspirant has astringents in its ingredients that help reduce pore size and thus help stop perspiration. Deodorants kill odor-causing bacteria. The trend in natural cosmetics seems to be toward deodorants, as they do not interfere with the body's natural release of moisture. The product you choose to use as a deodorant or antiperspirant is a matter of personal preference. We are all made just a little bit different, so you need to use a product that makes you feel your best. I have listed here a few of my favorite ingredients that have been proven to be effective as deodorants. Try them out. Perhaps you'll find a natural alternative that works just as well for you as your current remedy. You may also add them to after-bath splashes, powders, and creams.

Lovage: Lovage is a celery-scented herb with dark green leaves. It has cleansing and deodorizing properties. The seeds, leaves, and roots may be steeped in boiling water for a refreshing body wash. An effective antiperspirant can be made by covering the fresh leaves with brandy or vodka and letting it sit for a few weeks, then straining. Pregnant women and those with kidney problems should not use this plant, as it is a strong diuretic.

Witch hazel: This has long been my grandmother's favorite botanical antiperspirant. Witch hazel can be used alone or as a base for other products. If you find it is too drying you may want to mix a bit of vegetable glycerine with it. I also like to give my witch hazel a pleasant scent with a drop or two of a favorite essential oil.

Citrus peels: If you have ever taken a fresh piece of orange or lemon peel and smelled its fresh, clean scent you can see why these fragrant fruit skins make the perfect scent for a deodorant product. Let your fresh peels sit in some vodka or witch hazel for a few weeks. Then strain and use the liquid all over your body for a light and fresh clean scent. The citric acid from the peels also helps combat harmful bacteria on your skin's surface.

Rosewater: This lovely smelling product is naturally astringent and soothing to the skin. Rosewater is an age-old beauty product that has a number of uses. Mixed together with a bit of baking soda (use ½ cup rosewater and 1 teaspoon baking soda) it can be used all over the body as a safe and natural deodorant product. You may purchase rosewater or make your own (see page 260 for recipe).

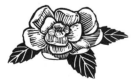

Cayenne Pepper Ointment

Christopher Columbus is credited with introducing cayenne pepper to Europe. He brought it back from the New World after one of his explorations of the tropical Americas. Cayenne comes from the Greek word meaning "to bite." It adds heat and bite to both culinary and cosmetic products. Capsaicin is the chemical found in hot peppers that gives them this heat. Not just for your favorite spicy dish, this substance is often used to treat those suffering from arthritis and rheumatism. Added to the bath or made into creams and ointments, it boosts circulation and warms your muscles.

1 small cayenne pepper, chopped
    with seeds
½ cup vegetable oil
2 tablespoons grated beeswax

In a small microwave-safe dish or saucepan combine the pepper with the oil and heat gently but do not boil. Let this mixture sit until cool. Strain and discard the pepper and seeds. Add the beeswax and heat again until the beeswax is melted. Stir well and spoon into a clean container. To use: Massage a small amount into your muscles and joints. If you desire a cream with a thinner consistency, add more vegetable oil and reheat. Note: Be careful when working with peppers not to touch your eyes. Wash your hands thoroughly with soap and water after handling.

Garden Note: To avoid damaging your plant never pull your peppers off when they are ripe. Instead, cut them off with a pair of sharp garden shears or scissors.

Yield: 4 ounces

Natural Sunscreen

¼ teaspoon borax powder
½ cup hot strong tea (use 2–3
   regular tea bags such as black
   or orange pekoe varieties and
   strain well)
¼ cup dark sesame seed oil
¼ cup avocado oil
1 tablespoon grated beeswax

This is a recipe for my basic, natural sunscreen. I would not recommend it for fair-skinned individuals or those people who sunburn quite easily. However, if your tan is well established or your skin does not require strong protection, this simple cream may do the trick. It contains dark sesame seed oil and avocado oil, both known for their sun-screening and skin-beautifying qualities. The tannic acid in the black tea also helps block harmful ultraviolet rays from the sun.

Dissolve borax in the tea, stir well, and set aside. Mix together oils and beeswax in a glass measuring cup. Place oil/beeswax in glass cup in a pan of water (1–2 inches of water) to make a water bath. Heat oil/beeswax in water bath over medium heat until beeswax is melted (8–10 minutes), stirring occasionally. When

---

SHADE TREES

If you find yourself outside without any sun protection, stand under a tree. Trees in full leaf provide protection from the sun and screen out harmful UV rays. In Durham, England, a study was done that measured the SPF protection of trees. Among the findings, it was discovered that an average single tree like an oak provides an SPF of 10–20. The more leaves on the tree the better; elms and sycamores offer an SPF of 30, and if you find yourself in the middle of a pine forest the SPF is well over 100. Take cover under a good tree — the darker the shade the better — spread out a blanket, and relax. You're protected.

the wax is melted, remove the mixture from the water bath. Slowly add the tea to the oil/beeswax, stirring briskly. (You can also put the mixture in the blender and whip.) Pour the lotion into a clean container and cool completely. Smooth this lotion onto your face and body before going out into the sun and reapply every hour during your time outdoors.

Yield: 8 ounces

Growing Loofah Sponges

*W*henever I give a talk or demonstration I always bring along a homegrown loofah (some spell it "luffa") sponge. People are surprised and delighted to learn that they can grow these body scrubbers in the garden, that they do not originate in the sea like their distant animal cousin, the sea sponge. These vegetable body brushes are easy and fun to grow and no garden beauty book would be complete without them!

The loofah belongs to a large family of plants that includes gourds, squashes, pumpkins, cucumbers, and melons. Loofahs are most closely related to cucumbers in appearance and growing habits. You can find loofah seeds in the seed section of many garden shops or by mail order from sources that specialize in unusual vegetables.

Once you have them, loofah seeds are easy to work with. They are large, flat, black seeds, much like a watermelon seed in appearance. Because of their large size, even small children can easily plant them. They sprout into a rambling vine that loves to climb in full sun. Choose a sunny location next to a fence, or use a trellis. You can also grow loofahs in containers with tomato cages or a wire trellis so the vines have somewhere to climb.

Loofah plants are sensitive to cold. You may want to start the seeds inside and move them outside when all danger of frost is past. Loofahs like soil that is rich in organic material or humus, so plant the seeds ¾–1 inch deep and cover with another inch of compost or manure.

Water your loofahs daily until the plants are established at 2–3 inches high. Then, water them deeply every 7 days. Fertilize the vines when yellow flowers appear. Loofahs grow vigorously and are similar in appearance to cucumber vines. The vegetable that will become the sponge is green, smooth, and even looks like a large cucumber. You can have as many as 25 loofahs on a single vine and each of them can reach 18 inches in length and weigh up to five pounds. Some people like to remove all of the first flowers from the vine and harvest the loofahs from the second blooms. They feel this produces a higher quality of sponge. You may want to try this.

Allow the loofahs to ripen on the vine until the skin turns dark yellow or brown. After picking, soak them in a bucket of water to soften the brown outer skin. Peel off all the brown skin. Remove the seeds and let dry. Store the seeds for next year's crop. After removing the peel and seeds let the "skeletons" of the loofahs dry in the sun. These fibrous skeletons are your sponges.

If you haven't discovered it already, I'll tell you now that loofahs are excellent exfoliators. Gently rubbing the loofah over your wet skin removes dead skin cells and surface dirt. Using a loofah is also excellent for your circulation and gives your skin a healthy glow.

Your loofahs will last quite a long time, but you must be sure to keep them clean and dry in between uses. To further discourage bacteria from growing you can clean the sponge using a 10 percent solution of bleach and water. Soak the sponge in the bleach solution and allow to dry. It is also a good idea to throw out your used sponges every couple of months.

HEALTHY SKIN CARE GARDEN

Plant a simple garden with everything you need for healthy skin. Choose sunflowers to gently scrub and cleanse the face, cucumbers, tomatoes, and potatoes to cleanse and soothe, and a border of herbs that are key ingredients in so many products and treatments. Now, what would a garden be without flowers? Plant geraniums, roses, honeysuckle, and lavender as well. All of these can be grown in either containers or a simple garden plot, except for the sunflowers, which really do better in the ground. The cucumbers and honeysuckle like to climb, so you can construct a simple trellis for them (I made one out of an old ladder) or plant them next to a fence, so they have something to hang on to. You will need a sunny location for your garden and a source of water nearby. Enjoy your pocket garden, which is full of bright colors and fresh scents. Not only will your complexion glow with health from its bounty, but your spirits will instantly be lifted when you look out upon this lovely patch, especially when the sunflowers bloom!

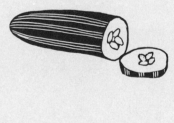

Massage and Relaxation

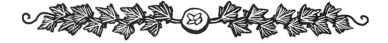

Gardening and relaxation to me are synonymous. Sure, gardening is often hard, dirty work mixed with some real frustrations, as any gardener will tell you who has lost a newly sprouted crop to frost or a herd of snails. But the benefits far outweigh the occasional heartbreak. Gardening is an interest—or rather a lifestyle—that can be enjoyed the rest of your life as a creative process that employs both your imagination and body.

The garden is the perfect spot to daydream, meditate, and visualize. It is where I go to get my creative juices flowing. Whether I am writing a magazine article or coming up with a solution to a family issue I find time spent among my growing plants is helpful. Sometimes I take notes and other times I just let my mind loose to wander. Some of my friends read in their gardens, practice simple meditation, and find it a wonderful spot to exercise. (Not that weeding, planting, and pruning don't provide enough!) You may also want to pick up a book on yoga and practice a few new positions in a quiet spot outdoors.

Today more and more people are enjoying the wonders of massage therapy or therapeutic touch. Once considered an indulgence for the rich and famous, massage is now becoming a part of our everyday lives. Millions of people all over the world practice one form or another of massage in their own homes. Look in your local telephone directory yellow pages and you will be amazed at the number of massage therapist listings. On a recent trip, I was delighted to see massage bars in several airports. One of my corporate fast-track friends tells me that in her building massages can be booked for quick 10-minute sessions in your own office.

Massage comes in many different forms, from Swedish to shiatsu. Whatever form you choose to practice, you'll find it is a wonderful way to relax and revive yourself. Anyone who has ever been given a massage knows what a wonderful feeling it can bring! Move your massage table or mat outdoors for a change. Under the shade of a large tree on a warm afternoon, a good massage will touch all of your senses and give you added energy. There are also several simple massage techniques that you can do all by yourself. Foot, hand, and scalp massages and simple neck rolls are all easy to give and perform solo. (See page 238 for a few basic steps to get you started.)

In this section I have also included recipes for several oils and lotions that you may use to enhance the experience. Two of my personal favorites that call for fresh garden herbs are Tranquil Breezes on page 244 and Modern Meditation Oil on page 248.

Scents are often used in both meditation and massage. This ancient practice of aromatherapy is very effective in changing both your physical and mental state. The use of scents in daily life and ceremonial rituals has been practiced for centuries by almost every civilization. Today aromatherapy products are found in a number of places, from high-priced natural beauty boutiques to the local grocery store. In fact, on a recent trip to the Oregon coast, my husband and I were in a small local grocery store, when over the loudspeaker an announcement was made that "all aromatherapy bath products are now on sale in aisle eight." People responded and began to move toward the designated grocery aisle. It was at that point that I realized natural products and treatments were truly becoming mainstream. What a beautiful discovery!

Relaxation techniques have long been used to fight headaches and muscle pain. Massaging the back of your neck can work as well as aspirin for easing headache pain. This is due to the connective muscles at the base of our necks that transfer tension from the spinal cord to the brain.

Massage and meditation techniques are also a great way to treat your skin. A clear head equals a clear complexion. Stress can cause our hormones, emotions, and oil glands to erupt, causing our skin to break out. Learning to take time out for yourself and to really relax benefits not just your mind and body but your skin as well. Create a spot in your garden or home for total relaxation. Take five to ten minutes each day and go to your special place. Sit or lie down, breathe deeply, and relax. You may feel silly at first, but you will have more energy and the condition of your skin and hair will noticeably improve.

Zen is a word from an Asian philosophy often used to describe someone or something that is incredibly calm and balanced. The goal of Zen is to become more enlightened by becoming aware of the unity of nature, the present moment, and who you are. Try the recipe for Zen Oil on page 241 to help you embrace this worldview. Zen gardens are another way to experience this. They are made up of a few elements that are so simple that they allow your mind to clear and exist in the moment. It may sound a bit too easy—but I think there may be something to be said for this ancient practice of sitting quietly, doing nothing, and watching the grass grow all by itself. Try it!

Massage oils and lotions are oil-based and have a long shelf life. They should be kept in a cool, dark location. Tinted bottles and jars are best since light can sometimes weaken their scent or cause the oils to spoil over time. If you suspect a product has gone bad it is best to discard it and mix up a fresh batch. Pouring your oils, lotions, and alcohols into clean hands is the best way to use them. This prevents contamination and the introduction of foreign ingredients.

Mae West was famous for saying, "Too much of a good thing is wonderful." I agree, especially when it comes to something like massage, so relax and enjoy yourself!

How to Give a Great Massage

THE BASIC MOVES:

One of the world's most popular forms of massage is Swedish massage. Here are the five basic strokes used. Keep in mind that you may incorporate these moves into your own unique form.

Glide: This is the basic stroke of any massage, and you may also hear it referred to as "effleurage." Using the palm of your hand, massage the body with strong, flowing strokes. This move gets the blood and lymph fluids circulating.

Rub: This move is also known as "friction." It consists of small back-and-forth motions using both hands. You may also try up and down, side to side, or circular motions. Unlike gliding, it is a small, even stroke and is meant to increase circulation and create heat.

Knead: This is a stimulating stroke. Treating the skin like bread dough, lift and release it. Kneading works best on thick parts of the body, such as the calves, thighs, and upper arms. It is used to stimulate the nervous system, gently stretch the muscles, and is a great way to warm up the body before exercising.

Vibrate: This move is done with the fingers. Shake, jiggle, or lightly tap the skin all over. Done quickly this can be invigorating; done slowly it can be quite relaxing.

Pound: This is usually done at the end of a massage. It is really more of a light drumming than a pounding and is meant to refresh the recipient. Use a cupped hand and gently pound or drum all over the recipient's body.

With these moves in mind, here are the five basic steps for giving a great massage:

1. First, choose a massage oil or lotion recipe or simply use a favorite light oil, such as sunflower, almond, or olive. You may add a drop or two of a selected essential oil to your oil or lotion for a bit of aromatherapy.

2. Locate a place for your massage. Choose a firm, steady surface. Beds are really not such a good location since soft mattresses absorb most of the impact of your massage strokes, stealing the benefits from your body. A massage table is ideal, but you can also use a futon, yoga mat, or layers of quilts and blankets on the floor. Make sure the environment is relaxing—no bright lights overhead or loud noises. Soft music is a nice option.

3. Massage is a physical activity for the giver as well as the recipient. Study the basic moves, keeping your strokes smooth and flowing. Avoid any sudden moves or interruptions. Keep your stroking toward the heart, not away from it. Your veins have little valves in them that keep the blood flowing toward the heart; you can cause damage to them if you are pushing them in the opposite direction.

4. Take your directions from your partner for areas that feel good or need special attention. Massage is like any other relationship in that it requires communication.

5. After the massage, linger and relax. Listen to a favorite song, read a book, or share a relaxing beverage. Savor the moment.

Stop and Smell the Roses!

1/4 cup grapeseed oil
1 tablespoon jojoba oil
1/2 tablespoon dried rosebuds and petals
1–2 drops scented rose oil (optional)

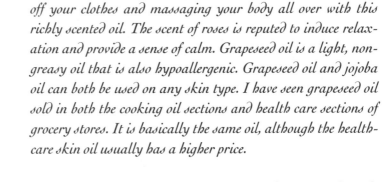

There is no stress-release program quite so effective as peeling off your clothes and massaging your body all over with this richly scented oil. The scent of roses is reputed to induce relaxation and provide a sense of calm. Grapeseed oil is a light, non-greasy oil that is also hypoallergenic. Grapeseed oil and jojoba oil can both be used on any skin type. I have seen grapeseed oil sold in both the cooking oil sections and health care sections of grocery stores. It is basically the same oil, although the health-care skin oil usually has a higher price.

Mix together all ingredients and gently warm the oil. This can be done in the microwave for 20–30 seconds or by placing your container in a warm water bath. Do not boil. Let the mixture sit for one week; do not strain. To use: Pour a small amount into clean hands and massage into your skin.

Garden Note: Use this simple solution to control black spot and powdery mildew on your roses. Mix 1 gallon of water with 1 tablespoon of baking soda, 3 drops liquid dish detergent, and 3 drops of vegetable oil. Mix well and spray on the tops and bottoms of the infected plant's leaves or stems. Keep the area under your plants clean, removing any diseased leaves that may have fallen to the ground.

Yield: 3 ounces

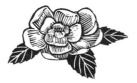

Zen Oil

"What is the sound of one hand clapping?" This is a deliberately irrational question that is used in the practice of Zen to evoke thought and reflection. This ancient practice is so popular today that it is used to define almost everything from flower arranging to baseball. I even saw "Zen soaps" sold in a bath catalog. This is my recipe for a scented massage oil that will help center your body, mind, and spirit. It contains ylang-ylang for energy, lavender for peace, and olive oil for wisdom.

½ cup light olive oil
1 tablespoon dried lavender flowers
1–2 whole clove buds
2–3 drops lavender essential oil
2–3 drops ylang-ylang essential oil

Place the lavender flowers inside a clean bottle or jar. Pour the olive oil over the lavender and add the drops of essential oils. Place a stopper or lid on your container and gently shake to mix the ingredients. Let the oil sit for one week. To use: Pour into clean hands and massage into your skin. This is also a nice oil to massage into your temples to help you sleep at night.

Garden Note: Ylang-ylang or perfume tree, as it is sometimes called, is a large tree with glossy leaves and spicy jasmine-scented yellow flowers. These trees are native to Southeast Asia and Australia.

Yield: 4 ounces

Garden Note: I am an avid rock collector and have stashes of rocks all around my home. I use these rocks inside flower vases, as plant markers, as a decorative accent to potted plants, on top of fence posts, and to keep doors open. Start your own helpful rock collection.

Caribbean Island Oil

½ cup avocado oil
½ cup grapeseed oil
2 tablespoons peanut oil
Dried zest of one small orange
½ teaspoon ground nutmeg
1 small cinnamon stick
5–6 black peppercorns
2–3 clove buds

Located in the arm of the Caribbean Sea that is bordered by the West Indies and South America lies a group of islands whose clear blue water and fragrant island plants lure travelers from all over the world. This popular vacation spot is known for its spirited food, cheerful calypso music, and relaxed attitudes. Massage a bit of this spicy citrus oil into your warm skin for a relaxing island respite.

Place all ingredients into a clean, dry bottle and cover the lid. Shake gently to mix and let sit for one to two weeks for the ingredients to blend. You may strain the oil through paper coffee filters if you like. I often leave it unstrained, as I like the look of the dried ingredients floating in my oil. To use: Pour a small amount into clean hands and massage into your skin.

Garden Note: Just for fun, when drying citrus peels cut them into shapes such as circles, stars, or crescents. You may also wind long strips of peels around bamboo skewers. These dried spirals add a decorative touch to your scented oil products.

Yield: 8 ounces

Peace, Love, and Massage

Peace, love, and rock and roll" was a popular statement of the flower children of the '60s and '70s. It was these three elements that they believed were necessary for a happy existence. Patchouli has a deep, musky lingering aroma and was the perfume of choice during this time of "free love." Incense sticks were burned in bedrooms around the world. This scented oil is inspired by those smoky love potions. To set the mood play some soul music softly in the background. Songs such as John Lennon's "Instant Karma," Burt Bacharach's "What the World Needs Now Is Love," and anything by Marvin Gaye are all good sound choices.

1 cup light sesame oil
Dried zest of one small orange
3 black peppercorns
3 drops essential oil of patchouli
3 drops essential oil of sandalwood

Place all ingredients into a clean, dry bottle and cover with a lid. Shake gently to mix and let sit for 1–2 weeks so that the ingredients can blend. Strain the oil through paper coffee filters if you like. To use: Pour a small amount into clean hands and massage into your skin.

Garden Note: Patchouli is a highly aromatic green herb with flower spikes. It is grown mainly in Malaysia. Its oil is used in making incense and perfumes and also has antiseptic qualities. It's a good remedy for insect bites.

Yield: 8 ounces

Tranquil Breezes

½ cup grapeseed oil
1 tablespoon apricot kernel oil
2 tablespoons light sesame oil
½ teaspoon vitamin E oil
1 tablespoon dried lavender flowers
½ tablespoon dried geranium leaves
2 teaspoons dried chamomile daisies
2–3 drops essential oil of cypress
1–2 drops essential oil of patchouli

I love to sit outdoors on a warm summer evening and listen to the trees move in the warm evening breezes. The sound of their rhythmic swaying to and fro is soothing, tranquillizing. This sensation allows me to let all my cares and worries be carried away in the wind. This oil would be perfect for a full-body massage outdoors with the serene sounds of nature all around you.

Place the dried herbs inside a clean, dry bottle. Pour the grapeseed, apricot kernel, sesame, and vitamin E oils over them and add the drops of essential oils. Cover the opening and shake the contents gently. Let the mixture sit for 1–2 weeks. Strain through paper coffee filters and store in a clean bottle with a tight-fitting lid. To use: Massage a small amount into your skin. This oil may also be added to your bath by using 1–2 tablespoons.

Garden Note: Hang a wind chime in your garden for a soothing melody anytime there is a gentle breeze. Many garden and import stores have a wide range of chimes to choose from. You can even make your own using materials such as bamboo, driftwood, old silverware, small pieces of metal, and seashells.

Yield: 5 ounces

Saint-John's-Wort Oil

Saint-John's-wort (Hypericum) *is a fast-growing ground cover. It takes its name from St. John the Baptist because it usually begins flowering on his feast day, June 24. Today this herb is being hailed as the new "wonder" plant and a good natural substitute for the antidepression drug Prozac. In this recipe, the plant's bright yellow flowers are infused in olive oil making a therapeutic oil that focuses on the body, not the mind, as a remedy for easing muscle and joint pain.*

¼ cup fresh Saint-John's-wort
  flower heads
½ cup warm olive oil

In a clean, dry jar combine the flower heads and olive oil. Place your container in a warm, sunny location and let it sit for one week. Every 2 days strain the oil and replace the flowers with new ones. At the end of the week you should have a pale yellow oil. To use: Massage a small amount of this oil on your joints to relieve pain. For headaches a small amount may also be massaged on the forehead.

Garden Note: I mow down my Saint-John's-wort each fall. In the spring I am greeted with a healthy, thick green patch of new shoots. This also helps contain the plants, as they are quick to spread across your yard.

Yield: 4 ounces

Hindu Love Potion

2 teaspoons dried jasmine flowers
½ vanilla bean, split
3 whole clove buds
1-inch piece of cinnamon stick
1 cup light sesame oil

*J*asmine flowers are a Hindu symbol of love. Their scent is a mental stimulant that increases our brains' beta wave activity, signaling excitement. The warm, spicy, and slightly heady scent of this oil makes it the perfect potion for a romantic evening massage. If you do not have jasmine growing in your yard, use jasmine tea, made from the dried flowers.

In a clean glass bottle or jar place the jasmine, vanilla, cloves, and cinnamon stick. Pour the sesame oil over these ingredients and seal the top. Let the mixture sit for 1–2 weeks. You may leave the dried flowers and spices inside your bottle (the scent of your oil will continue to increase) or strain out the solids before using. To use: Massage into warm skin during massage or after bathing.

Garden Note: Perfume a corner of your yard or patio by planting a jasmine vine. This fragrant vine thrives in sun or partial shade. Collect the flowers in the morning from July to October and air-dry them for use year-round.

Yield: 8 ounces

When we lived in Australia, my husband and I purchased a massage oil that was the perfect blend of rosemary, frangipani, and lavender, all known for their relaxing properties. My husband, Ray, liked the scent of this oil, especially when I employed it for a full-body massage. Now, back home in the United States, I can no longer find this restful blend. I did come up with this homemade version that my husband calls "a remarkable and enjoyable reproduction."

Mix together all the ingredients and pour into a clean, dry container. To use: Massage a small amount into your skin during massage or after bathing.

Garden Note: Frangipani trees are some of the most beautiful in the world, with shiny green leaves and clusters of creamy pastel flowers. Their heady scent perfumes the air around them. These trees are also called plumeria, pagoda, or temple tree, depending on where they are grown. In the Pacific Islands these flowers are strung into fresh necklaces, or leis.

Yield: 3 ounces

Ray's Relaxation Blend

¼ cup light sesame oil
1 tablespoon avocado oil
1–2 drops essential oil of rosemary
2–3 drops essential oil of lavender
2 drops essential oil of frangipani

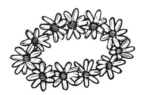

Modern Meditation Oil

¼ cup grapeseed oil
1 teaspoon dried clary sage leaves
1 teaspoon dried geranium leaves
5 drops essential oil of neroli
1 drop essential oil of narcissus

Meditation has risen in popularity and is fast becoming part of our modern-day lifestyle. Simple techniques, such as deep breathing, candle gazing, and self-hypnosis, are now practiced by executives, teenagers, and housewives. This road to lasting happiness and complete relaxation is being embraced by everyone. Many jobs are extremely stressful, creating the need for a mental oasis, a place we can go during the course of our day for peace. Massage a bit of this scented oil into your temples and at the base of your neck to strengthen your own meditative process.

Place the dried herbs inside a clean, dry bottle. Pour the grapeseed oil over them and add the drops of essential oils. Cover the opening and shake the contents gently. Let the mixture sit for 1–2 weeks. Strain through paper coffee filters and store in a clean bottle with a tight-fitting lid. To use: Massage a small amount into your temples and at the base of your neck. Now, focus your attention on an object and concentrate only on this object. Slowly count from 1 to 100, all the time maintaining your focus on that object. Close your eyes and try to imagine the object as clearly as possible. Sit calmly for 5–10 minutes. When you open your eyes you will feel totally relaxed and able to handle anything and anyone. Store your oil in a dark, dry location.

Garden Note: Clary sage is a hardy member of the sage family. It has green pointed leaves and pale purple or lavender flowers. Its strong scent is a powerful relaxant used to treat stress and fatigue.

Yield: 2 ounces

FLOWER MEDITATION

Traditionally called the thousand-petaled lotus meditation, this soothing exercise requires only a pen, a piece of paper, and your imagination. Pick a word that expresses a feeling you'd like to experience—like peace, for example. Write it down in the center of the paper and draw a circle around it; this will be the center of your flower.

Focus on the word and write down the next word or image that comes to mind, circling it to represent a petal on your flower. Don't worry if there is no clear relationship between the two words. Keep writing down the words that come into your mind and circling them around the center of your flower for at least 10 minutes, creating a beautiful flower of words and thoughts. When you are finished, carefully examine your paper—you may be surprised. The drawing before you may spark an idea about how to solve a problem or reveal your true feeling about some element of your life.

I focused on the word *energy* and realized by my writings and word selections that I needed to relax, focus on the big picture, and get more sleep. Spending time with family and friends was also important to me and a great way to recharge myself. See what wisdom your flower meditation brings you!

Venus's Massage Lotion

½ cup light olive oil
1 tablespoon dried marjoram leaves
¼ teaspoon vitamin E oil
1–2 drops essential oil of marjoram
    (optional)

The goddess Venus is believed to have created the herb marjoram and was the first to grow it. The sweet smell of its leaves is said to have come from her touch. This light lotion is a change from heavier massage oils and also makes a good all-over body moisturizer. Early Greeks enjoyed marjoram oil after bathing and used it to condition their hair and bodies.

Place your marjoram leaves in a clean, dry container. Mix together the olive oil and vitamin E oil and gently warm on the stove top or in the microwave; do not boil. Pour the warm oil over the dried herbs and let sit for 1–2 weeks. To strengthen the scent you may add a few drops of essential oil. Strain the mixture and pour into a clean bottle with a tight-fitting lid. To use: Massage a small amount into your skin. This recipe may also be used as a hair oil.

Garden Note: Plant marjoram in your garden to attract bees and butterflies.

Yield: 4 ounces

Gold Medal Oil

½ cup canola oil
¼ teaspoon vitamin E oil
1 teaspoon fresh ginger root juice
1 teaspoon dried thyme leaves
1–2 drops essential oil of lavender
1–2 drops essential oil of eucalyptus

Serious athletes all over the world believe in massage and its ability to soothe tired muscles. Ask any ardent competitor and he or she will tell you the importance of a good rubdown for soothing tired, overexercised muscles. Thyme, lavender, eucalyptus, and ginger are all warming and comforting to exhausted bodies. Use this massage oil to revive your body whether you are a weekend athlete or an Olympic contender.

Use a juice machine or blender to create the fresh ginger juice from ginger root. Mix together all the ingredients and pour into a clean bottle. Shake gently and let the mixture sit for a few days. You may strain the oil if you like. To use: Shake to remix the ingredients and pour a small amount into your hands. Massage the oil into your body, giving special attention to sore muscle areas.

Yield: 4 ounces

CANDLES

Lighting a candle creates immediate atmosphere that can transform a room, an event, a face. Candles symbolize peace, serenity, and warmth.

Fire and light have always fascinated man. Primitive torches made of dried branches dipped in suet may have been the first candles. Ancient Egyptian drawings depict burning flames; and archaeologists have found candlesticks that date as far back as 2500 B.C.

Today candles are very sophisticated and come in a variety of scents, shapes, and colors.

Here are a few of my favorite tips and techniques for using and enjoying candles outdoors in the garden. (Remember, never leave burning candles or melting wax unattended—they are both extremely flammable.)

- Make an easy outdoor candleholder by filling a flowerpot with sand. Set your candle in the center of the sand and light. To protect your flame on a windy day, cover the candle with an inexpensive glass hurricane.

- Place floating candles in birdbaths, pools of water, and ponds for a magical evening effect.

- To scent store-bought candles heat a metal skewer or large needle and make three holes at the base of the

(continued)

candle's wick. Place a few drops of scented oil inside each hole. Citronella or lemon grass oil is a popular choice for outdoor candles, as it keeps flying insects away.

- Burn a single, pretty candle when meditating. Focus on the burning flame and clear your mind of all thoughts.

- Make natural candleholders out of fresh greenery wreaths, flat rocks, large seashells, and garden statues.

- Line your pathways or patios with candles placed in jars or small paper bags filled with sand.

- Fresh vegetables also make fun candleholders. Simply hollow out sturdy ones, such as peppers, gourds, artichokes, or squash. Place a small candle inside and light.

PEACE OF MIND GARDEN

There are many old-fashioned herbal beliefs. One that intrigues me is that of a "healing" garden. It is believed that by choosing plants for their mind-balancing powers, you can create a special outdoor retreat that will heal whatever is troubling you and give you peace of mind.

Below I have listed a few plants and the qualities they are believed to accentuate. For example, if you desire more energy, try planting coriander, catnip, and red hollyhocks. By planting and tending to these plants you will receive added energy. Try using them in a favorite beauty recipe or making a small flower arrangement for your home or office.

Here are plant suggestions for your soothing garden spot:

Positive thoughts: basil, thyme, yarrow, hollyhock

Self-esteem boost: sunflower, clary sage, daisy

Extra energy: coriander, catnip, red hollyhock

Better sleep: Saint-John's-wort, chamomile, lavender

Increased communication: rose, calendula, snapdragon, cosmos

Improved health: tomato, cilantro, cayenne pepper

Increased intuition: mugwort, rose, Queen Anne's lace

Fragrance Products

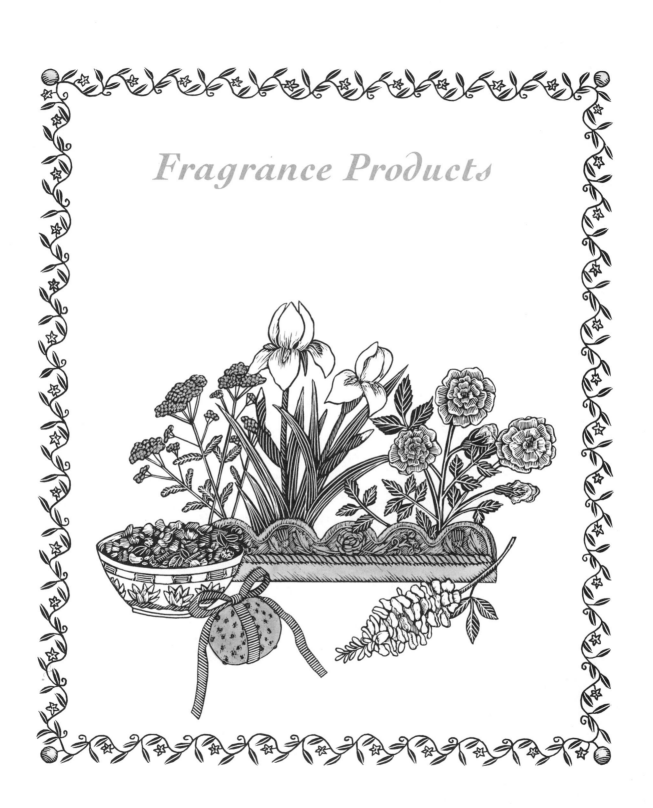

*I*t is hard to imagine a garden without fragrance. The scents and smells of the trees, plants, and flowers definitely enhance the outdoor experience. Garden sounds, colors, and sights are more enjoyable because we can smell the rich soil, aromatic herbs, and delicate flowers.

Fresh garden scents have the ability to change your state of mind, give you inner peace, and energize your whole body. This is where the concept of aromatherapy all began. We as humans cannot help but respond to scent. It captures our attention and can even alter our thought process.

Fragrance products to help soothe, calm, or invigorate are some of the easiest and most rewarding products to make. They do take a bit more time, since the mixtures need to sit for several weeks in order for their scents to develop. But your patience will be rewarded.

Creating your own scents is like writing a beautiful song or melody in which each individual ingredient is a note. This concept was developed in France, where people have long had a passion for fine perfumes. Septimus Piesse, a chemist, came up with the "note" idea of combining perfumes into harmonies according to the musical scale. He had three main categories: High notes are the first scent your nose detects and are usually bold, such as citrus. Middle notes determine the personality of the fragrance; these tend to be floral in nature. The low notes of a scent are those that linger on the skin or in your memories. The scent of vanilla is a popular low note used in commercial fragrances today.

The mystique surrounding fragrance has intrigued us since ancient times. Modern archaeologists have found paintings and drawings of early ceremonies that involved scented incense, candles, and oils. Cleopatra was rumored to scent the sails of her ship with rose oil to give her an aromatic advantage as she sailed into battle. She was a woman who knew what she wanted and used fragrance to get it.

Men also enjoy a good scent. Their fragrances tend to be bolder, spicier, more down to earth. A good one to try is the recipe for Saturn's Aftershave on page 266, inspired by the Roman god of agriculture.

All fragrance falls into six basic scent groups: floral, spice, wood, fruit, herbal, and exotic. Floral fragrances, such as rose, lavender, or carnation, tend to be relaxing, romantic, and give us a feeling of overall happiness. Spice scents, such as pepper, ginger, cinnamon, or clove, are comfortable, warming, and can also be energizing. Fruit scents, such as coconut, peach, apple, and strawberry, are light, uplifting, and fun to wear. Herbal scents, such as grass, rosemary, bay, basil, and pine, are reminiscent of the great outdoors. Exotic fragrances like sandalwood, vanilla, and ylang-ylang are more sophisticated and heavier. These latter fragrances tend to be the low notes in mixtures. Using these six basic groups, the combinations are almost endless.

There are several different types of fragrance products that you can make. Perfume, cologne, and aftershaves are similar in how they are made. The difference is in the percentage of alcohol used in relation to the amount of aromatic oil. Colognes and aftershaves usually contain less oil and are more inexpensive to create. The recipes in this section are closer to colognes than real perfume blends because real perfumes are very expensive to create. I have included a recipe for Solid Perfume on page 262 that is rich in scented oils. Alcohol-free scents, or "voiles," are becoming increasingly popular and are easy to make. These new light fragrances feel like a breath of fresh air next to your skin. Try the recipe for Bare Skin Mist on page 261. Body mists or splashes are another fun product to use. My mother enjoys using an after-bath product each morning. Because it is a lighter scent, she can splash it all over her body.

I have also included a few of my favorite potpourri recipes in this section. Potpourri has been used throughout history to scent the air and please the senses. I have it in just about every room of my house. I keep a small dish next to my bed for sweet dreams. In my closet I hang cedar and lavender sachets to ward off moths and other destructive pests. In the bath, I use it to scent my bathwater and freshen the air. I also have a wonderful small Sweet Bag necklace my daughter sewed for me that I often wear around my neck (see page 279 for directions). Potpourri is another way of preserving and enjoying favorite garden flowers and plants. You may also use it in beauty recipes, such as those for body scrubs, massage oils, and scented baths. I would not suggest using commercial potpourri in this fashion, as these are usually intended for decorative use and can contain dyes and other floral preservatives.

A garden can contain dozens of plants with fragrant leaves and petals. Some of them are predictable, such as mint, which smells as it should—minty. Others are wonderful surprises—witch hazel blooms in the winter with sweet-smelling flowers while tomato leaves have a fresh "green" scent (see recipe for Vine-Ripened Tomato Cologne on page 264). Take the time to observe and smell the many fragrant plants in your yard and neighborhood. You can even design and plant your own "fragrance garden." Use the plans on page 280 to get started.

Because fragrance products are made with alcohols and other scent fixatives they have a long shelf life. You can extend this by storing them in a cool, dark, dry location. Some of your scents may change over time as the ingredients continue to blend and develop. Try not to double the recipes unless you are making gifts. This ensures you will use up the product long before its scent has changed.

Fill your world with fragrance!

Attar of Roses

2–3 cups fresh rose petals and
    leaves
Coarse salt such as kosher or rock
    salt

*The fragrant petals of the damask rose (*Rosa damascena*) are the most commonly used in making attar of roses; however, you may also use any other strongly scented rose variety. Attar of roses is another name for the volatile oil contained inside the fresh petals and it is used in making rosewater and scented perfumes. Use only fresh unbruised petals that have been picked in the morning after the dew has evaporated but before the strong afternoon sun has warmed them.*

Gently wash the rose petals and leaves, and pat them dry between a layer of cotton towels or paper towels. Place a layer of the petals inside a clean ceramic crock or dark-colored glass jar. Over each layer sprinkle a thin covering of salt; repeat until the crock or jar is full. Cover your container tightly and place in a cool, dark spot for several weeks (3–6 weeks). The salt extracts the moisture from the petals and leaves, which should collect in the bottom of your jar. Strain the liquid through a coffee filter or several layers of cheesecloth. This is your scented attar of roses. To make fresh rosewater, add a drop or two of this oil to one cup of distilled water.

Garden Note: A good rule of thumb for watering roses is to water them deeply once a week in the morning. If you do this, it will encourage deeper roots, which will create stronger plants.

Yield: 1–2 ounces

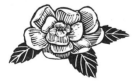

Bare Skin Mist

This is a lightweight fragrance that contains no alcohol, so it can be sprayed and spritzed all over your bare skin. You can even use it on your face and hair to refresh yourself throughout the day. It contains orange flower water, whose scent is from the bitter orange tree. This scent is also called neroli and is popular in many commercial products because it is believed to reduce stress. I purchase orange flower water at my local liquor store in the mixer section, but you may also find it in gourmet food stores.

¼ cup orange flower water
½ cup distilled water
½ teaspoon light sesame oil
1–2 drops peppermint oil

Stir together all ingredients and pour into a clean spray bottle. To use: Lightly spray the body mist all over your bare skin.

Yield: 6 ounces

Springtime Cologne

Take advantage of those first green sproutings in your garden by mixing up a batch of this floral cologne. After a long cold winter it is the perfect way to celebrate a change of season. The scent of both rose and lavender is famous for its calming effect. In fact, lavender has been proven by scientists to increase the brain's alpha-wave activity, which produces a state of relaxation.

2 tablespoons fresh rose petals
2 tablespoons fresh lavender flowers
1 teaspoon fresh lemon zest
1 tablespoon fresh rosemary leaves
1 tablespoon fresh mint leaves
1 cup water
1 cup vodka

Place the flowers, lemon zest, and herbs in a small saucepan and cover with the water. Heat the water gently for 5 minutes, but do not boil. Let the mixture cool completely, then add the vodka. Pour the entire mixture into a clean jar with a lid. Close the lid and place the jar in a cool, dry location for 2 weeks. Strain off all solids and pour your cologne into a pretty bottle with a lid or stopper. To use: Apply as you would any cologne or perfume.

Garden Note: Fresh mint leaves are a good remedy for insect bites. Simply rub a fresh leaf on the affected area.

Yield: 16 ounces

Solid Perfume

1 tablespoon beeswax
1 tablespoon almond oil
8 drops cologne or essential oil blend
    (see suggestions below)

*S*olid perfumes and scents have always been popular because they are long-lasting, easy to carry, and discreet—you can just rub them on and don't have to spray the air all around you. Throughout history great beauties such as Nefertiti, Cleopatra, Madame de Pompadour, and Irene Langhorne (the original Gibson Girl) carried their own personal scents, and now you can, too. They are easy to make and the procedures are basically the same as making a flavored lip balm. Pour your blends into vintage compacts or pillboxes for a unique package to slip into a pocket or purse. Any fragrance can be given a solid form—just remember that oil-based scents will last longer.

In a heat-resistant container or small saucepan, gently heat the beeswax and oil until the beeswax is melted. Stir in the scented oils or cologne and pour into a clean container with a lid. Allow the mixture to cool completely. To use: Rub your finger across the solid perfume and apply the scent to your pulse points or wherever you wish.

Yield: 1 ounce, 1–2 compacts

Scent suggestions:

> **Fruity:** 3 drops peach oil, 3 drops sweet orange oil, 2 drops chamomile oil
>
> **Spicy:** 3 drops clove oil, 3 drops sandalwood oil, 2 drops cinnamon oil
>
> **Exotic:** 5 drops vanilla oil, 3 drops ylang-ylang oil

Fresh Mowed Grass

The smell of just-cut grass transports everyone to a cherished childhood memory. Mine is when my father finally let me use our riding lawn mower. After months of hearing him explain to me how it was done and watching him demonstrate the proper mowing pattern to use, I was ready to do it myself. The big day finally came—when I finally climbed up on the mower it was a wonderful feeling of being grown up and doing an important outdoor chore. Many of my friends remember making daisy chains or rolling down a sloping lawn until they could not stand up straight. The fresh scent of this green cologne may recall your own childhood lawn memories.

2 tablespoons fresh-cut grass
1 teaspoon fresh chamomile daisies
1 teaspoon fresh clover flowers
¼ cup vodka
⅛ teaspoon castor oil

In a clean jar with a lid place all of the fresh ingredients. Pour the vodka and castor oil over them. Put the lid on your jar and shake gently. Set the jar in a cool, dark place for 1–2 weeks. Strain the liquid and test the scent. For a stronger scent add more fresh ingredients and wait another week. To use: Apply as you would any cologne product.

Garden Note: Mowing the lawn with an old-fashioned push-style mower is great exercise. I recently read a study that stated pushing a mower burns as many calories as low-impact aerobics, tennis, or downhill skiing. So trim your waist as you trim your lawn!

Yield: 2 ounces

Vine-Ripened Tomato Cologne

4 tablespoons fresh tomato leaves, chopped
1 tablespoon fresh lemon zest
1 teaspoon fresh basil leaves
1 teaspoon fresh mint leaves
1 cup vodka
¼ teaspoon glycerine

This cologne may seem a bit different at first, but think about it this way: What better inspiration for a fragrance product than the queen of the vegetable garden? Fresh plant leaves help make the ultimate summer scent. This cologne is light, fresh, alluring, and smells amazingly like a just-picked tomato — delicious!

Place all of the fresh leaves and lemon zest inside a clean jar or bottle. Pour the vodka and glycerine over them; shake gently. Cover the bottle top and let sit in a cool, dark spot for 2 weeks. Strain the liquid and discard any solids. Pour your cologne into a clean bottle with a tight-fitting lid. To use: Apply as you would any cologne product.

Garden Note: Tomatoes make wonderful, edible landscaping plants. They can be grown on trellises and come in a variety of lovely colors, such as white, yellow, purple, and orange, as well as the good old tomato red.

Yield: 8 ounces

Giverny Floral Water

For artist Claude Monet, gardening and painting were definitely connected. He once confessed, "I owe having become a painter to flowers." Monet was the leader in one of the most sweeping revolutions in the history of art—Impressionism. His unique use of muted colors and natural light and shadows gave us another beautiful way to view the world. My favorite paintings are those from his home and garden in Giverny, France. When I look at these great works I can hear the great artist saying his famous line, "I must have flowers always, always."

1 cup fresh rose petals
½ cup fresh wisteria blossoms
¼ cup fresh poppy petals
1 tablespoon fresh lavender flowers
1 cup distilled water
½ teaspoon dried orrisroot powder

In a small saucepan place the fresh flower petals and flowers and cover with the water. Heat gently, but do not boil. Simmer for 5 minutes, covered. Keep the pan covered and let the mixture cool completely. Strain the liquid and discard the flower solids. Stir in the orrisroot powder and pour the scented water into a clean bottle with a tight-fitting lid. To use: Apply as you would any cologne or after-bath splash.

Garden Note: For a Monet-style lawn, plant it with autumn crocus. In the summer, peel back small pieces of your lawn and plant the small bulbs. Lay the sod back down and water well. In the fall your lawn will bloom with color.

Yield: 8 ounces

Saturn's Aftershave

1 tablespoon fresh yarrow flowers
1 tablespoon fresh sage leaves
3 bay leaves
1 teaspoon dried cardamom seeds
5 black peppercorns
3 whole clove buds
½ cup vodka
½ cup witch hazel
1 teaspoon glycerine

In Roman mythology, Saturn is the Roman god of agriculture who fled from Mount Olympus and settled in Italy. There he established a golden age, in which all people were equal and harvests were plentiful. Ancient Romans held a seven-day festival in honor of this god, which was named the Saturnalia. This fresh scent full of harvested herbs and spices would have been perfect to wear during this time of unrestrained celebration.

Place all the fresh leaves and dried spices inside a clean jar or bottle. Pour the vodka, witch hazel, and glycerine over them; shake gently. Cover the bottle top and let sit in a cool, dark spot for 2 weeks. Strain the liquid and discard any solids. Pour your cologne into a clean bottle with a tight-fitting lid. To use: Apply as you would any aftershave or cologne product.

Garden Note: Yarrow is an old medicinal herb, supposedly used by Achilles to treat his wounded men in the Trojan Wars. It grows best in full sun. Cut your plants after the first flowers fade and they will bloom a second time.

Yield: 8 ounces

Famous for saying, "Never put off till tomorrow what you can do today," Thomas Jefferson was a great president and gardener. Monticello, his home in Virginia, with its well-planned colonial gardens is growing proof of this. He was a man who believed in democratic ideals and horticultural experimentation. Jefferson devoted many years to developing crops, such as olives and rice, that he believed would improve the living standard of American farmers. He once wrote, "The greatest service that can be rendered any country is to add a useful plant to its culture." This aftershave recipe is a tribute to a garden legend.

Place all the fresh flowers, leaves, and orange zest inside a clean jar or bottle. Pour the brandy, witch hazel, and glycerine over them and shake gently. Cover the bottle top and let sit in a cool, dark spot for 2 weeks. Strain the liquid and discard any solids. Pour your cologne into a clean bottle with a tight-fitting lid. To use: Apply as you would any aftershave or cologne product.

Garden Note: Colonial gardens were both practical and beautiful. Lavender was grown in almost every garden and was added to bath and laundry water because it was naturally antiseptic and smelled good. The word *lavender* comes from the Latin *lavre*, which means to wash.

Yield: 8 ounces

Monticello Aftershave

¼ cup hollyhock flowers
1 tablespoon lavender flowers
2 bay leaves
2 tablespoons orange zest
1 tablespoon thyme flowers
½ cup brandy
½ cup witch hazel
1 teaspoon glycerine

Hemingway's Havana Aftershave

Ernest Hemingway is one of the most famous and influential American writers of the twentieth century. This aftershave takes its inspiration from memorable scents found in Havana pubs that Hemingway was known to frequent. It is the perfect blend of anise, jasmine, and cedar.

1 cup light rum
1 tablespoon dried jasmine flowers
3–4 star anise seeds
3–4 drops essential oil of cedar
⅛ teaspoon castor oil

Mix together all ingredients and pour into a clean jar with a tight-fitting lid. Place the jar in a dark, cool place for 2 weeks. Strain the liquid and discard any solids. Stir in the castor oil as a scent fixative and pour into a clean cologne bottle. To use: After shaving, pour a small amount into your hands and pat on your face.

Garden Note: Spring-blooming jasmine makes a fragrant indoor vine. It grows easily around wire topiary frames available at many craft and garden shops.

Yield: 8 ounces

007 Skin Bracer

Everyone knows the number 007 belongs to Ian Fleming's superspy, James Bond. He is handsome, debonair, a fast driver, and incredibly cool. Bond has been saving the world for several decades with a "shaken–not stirred" attitude. Your man may not fight politically corrupt individuals for a living or search the world for lost microchips, but like 007, I am sure he will not turn down a bit of extra pampering, especially from a pretty woman. Mix up a batch of this exhilarating skin bracer for him to use after shaving and before his next secret assignment.

¼ cup Russian vodka (or any pure vodka)
¼ cup witch hazel
½ tablespoon fresh lemon zest
1 teaspoon camphor spirit

Mix together all ingredients. Let the mixture sit for a few days to allow the ingredients to mix and strengthen. Strain the liquid into a clean bottle with a tight-fitting lid. To use: Splash on the skin after shaving.

Garden Note: Camphor spirit comes from trees that grow in Java, China, and Brazil. It gives a cool feeling to your skin and is extremely refreshing.

Yield: 6 ounces

NATURAL INSECT REPELLENTS

Working outdoors will inevitably lead to encounters with flying and crawling insects. All gardens have good and bad bugs. They are constantly battling it out in your yard. Some of the beneficial ones found in your garden are dragonflies, ladybugs, and ground beetles. They feed on plant-destroying ones such as aphids, caterpillars, and spider mites. This is nature's way of keeping our environment well balanced. Bugs can also bug us. We all know how irritating a hungry mosquito is or how destructive a colony of ants can be.

Here are some natural and effective repellents you can try in an effort to make gardening a bit more comfortable.

Citronella: One of the most popular and common natural insecticides is citronella oil. I have seen it sold in candles, incense, lotions, and oils. Extracted from lemon grass, the oil has a lemony scent that repels insects. You may purchase the essential citronella oil and add a few drops to your favorite sunscreen or lotion. I also bought a citrosa plant at our local garden center last summer. It is actually a geranium but has the scent of citronella. Planted in a container or in the yard, the citrosa will help keep flying insects away.

Eucalyptus: Many flying pests, such as flies and mosquitoes, do not like the scent of these trees. They are often planted around fruit orchards to act as natural wind breaks and insect repellents. If you do not have a eucalyptus tree in your yard you may purchase scented Australian tea tree oil or essential oil of eucalyptus at many

(continued)

natural food stores. Mix a few drops of tea tree oil into a cup of water and spray the scented mixture onto your skin and hair. You may use this spray around the garden to help eliminate flying pests.

Mint: I love the scent of mint and always tuck a small bunch into my flower arrangements. Not only does mint provide my home with a clean fresh scent, it helps ward off ants and flies. Basil and bay leaves also work equally well.

Cloves and coffee grounds: Ants cannot stand the scent of either cloves or used coffee grounds, so sprinkle used coffee grounds around your plants. This will also help them grow better, as most plants can use a bit of acid added to their soil. You may use strong clove oil to rid your home safely of ants as well. For serious problems, make this lethal mixture to rid your home of ants: Mix together 2 cups of borax and 1 cup sugar and stir well. Sprinkle on ant trail or place in small containers.

Fleur-de-Lis Body Powder

Iris flowers are named after a goddess who used to ride rainbows, because they bloom in so many different colors. Their cultivation dates back to the Middle Ages. The French royal symbol, fleur-de-lis, is taken from the flowers of this elegant bulb plant. Orrisroot powder, which has been used for centuries in perfumes, potpourri, and powders as a fixative, comes from the roots of the white iris, Iris florentina. *The fine white powder has a delicate violet scent and can be found in many natural food stores and herb shops. You may also dry your own. Fresh orrisroot has only a faint fragrance, but when dried it becomes quite aromatic.*

1 tablespoon orrisroot powder
½ cup cornstarch

Place the two ingredients in a small glass bowl or jar and mix well. Store your powder in a dry container with a tight-fitting lid. To use: Apply with a powder puff or soft brush to dry skin.

Garden Note: Unlike other bulbs, iris bulbs or rhizomes do not like to be planted in the soil. Instead they prefer to lie on top of the ground. Only their roots go into the soil. If they are buried in the ground they may rot.

Yield: 4 ounces

Arabian Jasmine Powder

1 cup rice flour
1 tablespoon finely ground dried
    jasmine flowers
1 teaspoon sweet almond oil
1–2 drops essential oil of jasmine

Jasmine is a fast-growing vine with delicate, strong-scented flowers. Arabian jasmine, or pikake as it is also known, is what is used in popular jasmine tea blends, a highlight of any garden tea party. It is a featured plant in any scented garden design, used to provide privacy and shade. In this recipe dried flowers are finely ground and added to rice flour to make a rich body powder. Adding a bit of sweet almond oil to the mixture enhances the feeling of elegance the finished product has.

Place the rice flour in a bowl or resealable plastic bag. Add the jasmine flowers and oil and mix well. Pour the scented powder into a clean, dry container. To use: Massage into dry skin or use a salt or sugar shaker and sprinkle the powder all over your body.

Yield: 8 ounces

Victorian Geranium Powder

Scented geraniums were at their height of popularity during the early 1900s. Victorian garden catalogs feature over 200 varieties of these aromatic plants, with scents ranging from the common to the exotic. Today's garden catalogs also offer these fragrant members of the Geraniaceae family. Although they are not as prevalent as in my grandmother's time, it seems interest is growing in these old-fashioned flowers. This scented body powder is easy to make from fresh-cut leaves and will keep your body dry and comfortable.

1 cup cornstarch
6–8 fresh scented geranium leaves, washed and dried
1–2 drops essential oil of geranium (optional)

Place the cornstarch in a resealable jar or plastic bag. Add the fresh leaves and essential oil. Seal the container and gently shake to mix. Let the powder sit for 3–4 days, shaking the container once a day. Remove the leaves and discard. Pour the powder into a clean, dry container. To use: Sprinkle onto clean, dry skin or apply using a fluffy powder puff.

Garden Note: One of my favorite spots to place pots of scented geraniums is in my bathroom. I like to prune my plants while running my bathwater and toss the leaves directly into the tub. I enjoy the fragrance, and my plants grow healthy and strong.

Yield: 8 ounces

Chamomile Arrowroot Powder

½ cup arrowroot powder
1 tablespoon finely ground dried chamomile flowers
1–2 drops essential oil of chamomile (optional)

*A*rrowroot powder is made from the tropical arrowroot plant. This tall plant has spear-shaped, very shiny green leaves. The fine white, starchy powder is used as a thickener in cosmetics products. It comes from the dried rhizome found at the plant's base near its roots. It also makes an excellent body powder when mixed with dried chamomile. You can purchase arrowroot powder at the grocery or natural food store.

Place the arrowroot powder in a bowl or resealable plastic bag. Add the chamomile flowers and oil and mix well. Pour the scented powder into a clean, dry container. To use: Massage into dry skin or apply with a powder puff after bathing.

Garden Note: An old belief is that chamomile was the garden's doctor. When planted near sick or dying plants it seemed to cure them and make them grow again.

Yield: 4 ounces

Elizabethan Pomander

2 small whole oranges
2 teaspoons orrisroot powder
½ cup whole clove buds

*E*lizabethan ladies made scented pomanders out of fruits and spices and wore them on chains around their neck or attached to their girdles. These prized, scented charms gave them an alluring and pleasing scent. We have all grown up making the classic orange clove pomanders to hang in closets and give as gifts. Here are a few other combinations to try using apples, kumquats, lemons and limes, and a variety of spices. Whether you wear them as the Elizabethans did, float them in the bath, or set them out in bowls to perfume the air in your home, this scented craft is fun to try and makes a lovely gift.

With a large needle or toothpick pierce holes in the skin of the orange to form a pattern. Swirls, circles, and initials are all fun to try. Take care not to make a straight line, as this could cause the skin of your orange to split. Place a clove bud inside each hole. After you have filled your fruit with cloves, roll the orange in the orrisroot powder. Place the orange in a warm, dry place and allow it to dry for 3–6 weeks. As the fruit dries, it will shrink, tightening up your pattern.

Yield: 2 small pomanders

Variations to try:

Using the basic technique outlined above try these simple variations:

Apple-cinnamon: Instead of orrisroot powder, roll your clove-studded apple in ground cinnamon.

Kumquats: These make cute mini-pomanders and can be worn as a necklace or added to a bowl of potpourri. Instead of orrisroot powder, roll the tiny clove-studded fruits in ground allspice berries.

Lemon, lime: Instead of oranges, try other citrus fruits such as lemons and limes. Roll the clove-studded fruits in ground nutmeg.

Holiday Potpourri

4 cups dried pine needles
1 cup pine cone scales or small pine cones
1 cup juniper berries or holly berries
2 cups cinnamon sticks broken into small pieces
½ cup dried orange peel
2 tablespoons clove buds

*M*aking this dry potpourri blend is a festive holiday tradition. Start by taking a hike or walk in a nearby wooded area or forest. As you are exercising and breathing in the freshly scented air, gather fresh evergreen branches, pine cones, woodland berries, and other aromatic ingredients for your own holiday blend. Once home, dry your fresh ingredients in a warm oven and enhance their natural scents by adding some dried citrus peels and spices. Place a large container full of this mixture next to your fireplace. The heat from the flames will warm the mixture, releasing its woodland scent. You can also throw a handful into the fire and watch the flames dance. Packaged in a decorative container it makes a lovely hostess present to take to holiday parties.

(For information on drying fresh ingredients, see page 26.) In a large bowl mix together all ingredients and stir well. You may add more ingredients until the mixture has the look, scent, and texture you desire. Store your potpourri inside an airtight container. To refresh the scent you may add a few drops of scented pine or clove oil. To use: Set out in shallow bowls around your house or toss approximately ½ cup into a burning fire.

Yield: 8 cups (64 ounces)

In the winter when there are not as many fresh flowers and leaves to scent my home and freshen the air I like to use this blend of household spices. It has a warm, uplifting scent that, when simmered on your stove top, gives your house a cozy feel. It also helps add humidity to the air. During the winter months colder temperatures and household heating reduces the amount of humidity in the air. This dry air affects the condition of our skin and hair, both of which need moisture to stay healthy.

1 cup cinnamon sticks, broken into small pieces
4 whole nutmeg seeds
½ cup star anise seeds
½ cup cardamom pods
½ cup whole allspice berries
½ cup dried orange peel (you may also use grapefruit or lemon peel)
2–3 drops essential oil of clove (optional)

Mix together all the ingredients in a large bowl. Pour into an airtight container. To use: Add ¼ cup of potpourri to 4 cups (one quart) of water. Heat gently on low heat on your stove; do not boil. You may add more water if needed.

Garden Note: Cinnamon trees have shiny green leaves with creamy white flowers and dark blue berries. Cinnamon sticks are made from the tree's dried bark. These trees are native to Sri Lanka, but can be grown in other tropical climates.

Yield: 3 cups (24 ounces)

Cedar Closet
Sachets

Cedar has been used for years to line clothes closets, drawers, and chests. The wood from the fragrant cedar tree is a proven repellent to fabric-destroying pests. These sachets are small scented sacks that can be used to keep your clothes and linens pest-free and sweet-smelling. I like to use a combination of lavender and cedar shavings. If you do not have access to nature's supply of fresh wood shavings, an excellent source is pet shops, where they are often sold in bulk as a pet's bedding material.

½ cup cedar wood shavings
½ cup dried lavender flowers

Mix together the cedar and lavender and fill small muslin tea bags or tie into bundles using old cotton handkerchiefs. To use: Hang in closets or place inside drawers. You will need to change these sachets each year since the scent will fade over time.

Garden Note: If you have a large shade tree in your yard, place a garden seat or bench under it. This makes a wonderful spot to relax or read a good book.

Yield: 1 cup, approximately 2–3 sachets

Bedside Potpourri

1 cup dried lavender flowers
1 cup dried rosebuds or dried rose petals
1 vanilla bean
½ cup dried chamomile flowers
½ cup dried jasmine flowers
2–3 drops of essential oil of lavender or chamomile (optional)

This mixture combines my favorite summer garden flowers in a relaxing potpourri that is perfect for the bedroom. Fill a crystal vase with this mixture and keep it next to the bed. You can even sprinkle a bit under your pillows for sweet dreams! If you forgot to save your flowers this past summer, don't worry. Many natural food stores have a wide selection of dried flowers and herbs.

Using a pair of scissors cut the vanilla bean into small pieces. Mix together all the ingredients in a large bowl. For a stronger scent add the essential oil and stir well to mix. Pour into an airtight container for storage. To use: Place in a shallow dish next to your bed or tie some up inside a pretty lace handkerchief and tie with a satin ribbon.

Yield: 3 cups (24 ounces)

Sweet Bags

*I*n Europe during the sixteenth century "sweet bags" consisting of scented herbs and flowers were worn or carried as a type of personal potpourri. My daughter Lauren created her own version of this custom by sewing together two simple felt shapes and filling the little bag with dried herbs and flowers. These tiny pillows can be made into pins or necklaces and make lovely gifts.

1–2 tablespoons dried herbs or
    flower petals
Pinch orrisroot powder (optional)

Draw a small, simple shape such as a heart or circle on a piece of felt. Cut out two shapes and stitch together, leaving a small opening. Fill the pillow with herb or flower petals and stitch closed. Attach a long ribbon, for a necklace, or pin backing to the felt. You may also wish to decorate your sweet bag with embroidery, beads, or buttons.

Yield: 1 sweet bag

FRAGRANCE GARDEN

Growing plants with sweet flowers and aromatic foliage increases your enjoyment of your garden. A plant's fragrance has the ability to change your state of mind, by making you feel more relaxed or alert. Our bodies cannot help but respond to scent, and outdoors in the garden is no exception. Even the most delicate fragrance captures our attention.

Plant your own personal fragrance garden. Try not to include too many scents, as this may be overwhelming to your sense of smell. Instead, choose a few complementary scents or plants that bloom in different seasons for a year-round effect.

Here are a few of my favorite scented plants to plant in your own yard and use in making scented beauty products:

Vines: Scented vines can be used to create small "aromatherapy rooms" or screens in your garden. Try planting honeysuckle, jasmine, and wisteria.

Trees: A large, scented tree can perfume your whole yard and provide you with cool shade on hot summer days. Magnolia, mimosa, orange, and linden trees all have fragrant blossoms.

Night Flowers: A scented night garden can be quite enjoyable, especially for gardeners who work away from home during the day. By planting night-blooming plants, you can enjoy their scent in the evening when you get home. Plant evening primrose, four o'clocks, moonflowers, hostas, and night-scented stocks.

Herbs: Most herbs have a unique scent, especially when you rub up against them or pinch off a leaf or two. Try different varieties of mint, sage, basil, rosemary and lavender. These are all well known for their scents.

Flowers: The scent of certain flowers can bring to mind vivid and special memories for many of us. Whenever I smell a gardenia, I think of my grandmother, as this is her favorite scent. When my lilies-of-the-valley bloom, it is my wedding day that comes to mind. Plant some favorite scents and recount your own pleasant fragrance memories. Try roses, lilies-of-the-valley, carnations, peonies, day-lilies, and gardenias.

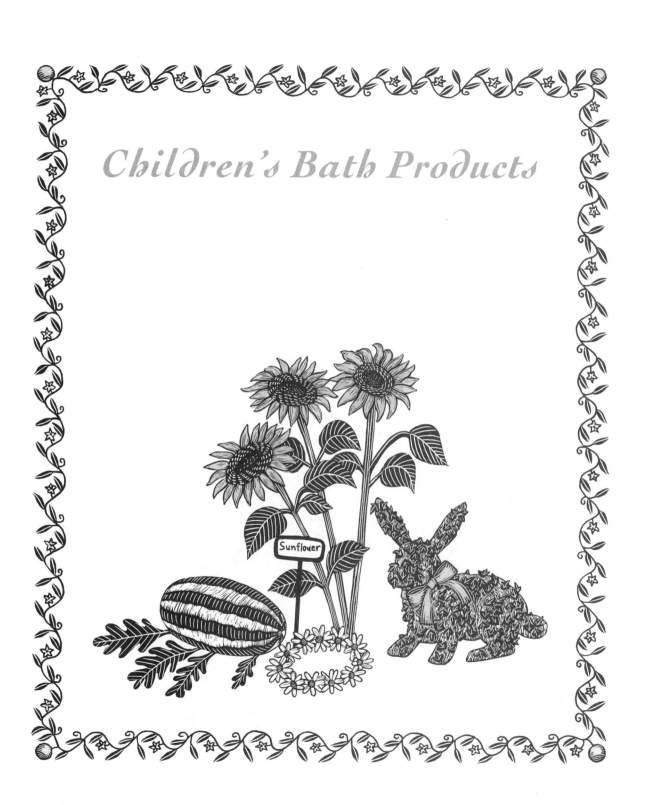

Children's Bath Products

Sunflower

Many of my favorite books growing up contained gardens — Winnie the Pooh and his friends had the Hundred Acre Woods, Beatrix Potter's books had wonderful English garden scenes. My all-time favorite childhood book was Frances Hodgson Burnett's *The Secret Garden*. It was the ultimate tale of botanical fantasy. I still get excited whenever I read the part where Mary finally finds the key and unlocks the garden door. Both my husband and I have read the story to our daughters several times. My older daughter, Lauren, wants us to turn her room into the secret garden, complete with an ivy-covered door. Many of these literary gardens, along with my own childhood garden memories of lavender wands (see page 298), flower crowns (see page 295), and wonderful bubble baths, were the inspiration for the recipes in this section.

Children's bath products vary from adult products in that young people have finer hair, sensitive skin, and more delicate noses. Strong scents and ingredients are not appropriate for immature systems. Instead, lightly scented products containing pure, natural ingredients are best for cleaning and moisturizing skin and hair. It is important to keep children's skin clean, dry, and fresh. Doing this will greatly reduce the risk of skin problems or rashes that some children can develop.

Bathing should also be fun. If you make it something your child wants to do, you help your children develop good health habits. My girls know better than to go to bed with dirty skin and hair. Making bath time enjoyable seems to take some of the chore out of it. I encourage their own bathing ideas and have included them in this section. Check out Lauren and Marie's Cooking Bath recipe on page 290 for some bath time fun.

Many of the recipes and projects in this section are so easy to create. Children can make them along with their parents, although very young children may need more help. They also make wonderful presents for birthdays and holidays. Mix up a batch of Scented Play Dough on page 297 to take to a friend's celebration.

I have also included a few entertaining and educational gardening projects to try with your children. Last summer, my daughters and I planted the Home Sweet Sunflower Home on page 303. It grew and became one of their favorite "secret" spots. We also learned a bit about birds as they attacked and ate our flower home in the fall! Children's gardens are meant to be enjoyed and played in. They should be full of color and scents. It is also a good idea to plant a few treats, such as cherry tomatoes, strawberries, and chocolate mint, which can be nibbled on and enjoyed during a teddy bear tea party or a quiet moment spent reading a good book.

Children's bath products should be stored in clean, nonbreakable containers. It is always best to keep any cosmetic product, even natural ones, where children cannot get into them. Something that smells good is often a temptation and could upset a small stomach if ingested.

Childhood is all about enjoying yourself and having fun. I always tell my daughters that life is meant to be lived and their job is to be the best at it!

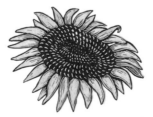

Watermelon Bath Splash

Watermelons are fun for children to grow. They have easy-to-handle big black seeds and love to be watered—sometimes twice a day. This fresh-scented bath splash is fun to use, especially during the warm summer months. You can make fresh watermelon juice by processing the watermelon in a blender or food processor and straining. (Mixed with a bit of club soda it makes a refreshing summertime drink.) Watermelon juice contains a high amount of vitamins A, B, and C, all of which keep skin healthy and glowing.

¼ cup fresh watermelon juice
2 tablespoons witch hazel
½ cup distilled water

Combine the watermelon juice, witch hazel, and water. Pour into a clean container. To use: Splash onto your child's body or pour into a clean spray bottle and let your child do the spraying after bathing. For a longer shelf life, store any remaining splash in the refrigerator.

Garden Note: Watermelons originally come from the African tropics. If you live where summers are long, hot, and humid they will thrive. If not, I would start my melons indoors to give them a jump-start on the growing season.

Yield: 6 ounces

Strawberry Shortcake Bath

½ cup fresh strawberries (you may
    use frozen)
½ cup heavy cream
2 cups water
1 tablespoon cold-pressed castor oil

This is a rich, fruit-scented bath that is perfect for dry, delicate skin. It makes the bathwater a creamy shade of pink and contains two natural emollients—fresh cream and castor oil. Castor oil has been used for years as a health tonic. It comes from the seeds of the castor plant. This oil is used in many bath products because it easily disperses through the bathwater rather than floating on top as other oils do. The heat from the warm water helps the oil penetrate and moisturize dry skin.

Place all of the ingredients into a blender and process on High until you have a smooth, creamy liquid. You may strain this mixture if you like. To use: Pour the strawberry mixture into a warm bath and stir well.

Garden Note: Pine needles make a good garden mulch (ground cover) for strawberry plants—a great way to recycle garden trimmings or old Christmas trees.

Yield: 24 ounces, enough for one bath

Tutti-Frutti Lip Gloss

1 teaspoon coconut oil
1 teaspoon petroleum jelly
1–2 drops selected fruit-flavored
    extract or oil

Mix up batches of these fruit-flavored lip glosses to tuck inside backpacks, coat pockets, and keep in bedside drawers. Little lips need protection, especially during the winter months. I like to use fruit-flavored extracts and oils from the grocery store. Some of the more exotic flavors, such as kiwi, can be found at gourmet cooking supply shops.

Mix together the coconut oil and petroleum jelly and stir well until smooth and creamy. Add the flavored extract with an eyedropper, one drop at a time. Stir well and spoon into a clean small jar or lip gloss container. To use: Spread on lips.

Give your children a small container or spot in your yard just for them. Let them plant whatever they like and care for it. Don't worry if they keep digging up the seeds to "check on them"—this is how many famous botanists started out.

Yield: ½ ounce

Tinkerbell's Magic Pixie Dust

Being a parent I often have to answer those hard questions like "What is a pixie?" Well, a pixie is a playfully mischievous elflike creature. The queen of all pixies would most certainly be Peter Pan's loyal friend, Tinkerbell. If you remember in that tale, Tink's magic dust is what made the children fly. This lightly scented powder isn't really magic, but when applied with a fluffy feather puff and a bit of imagination—it certainly seems to be.

1 cup cornstarch
1 tablespoon orrisroot powder
1 teaspoon finely ground, dried lavender flowers
1 teaspoon finely ground, dried rose petals
½ teaspoon gold glitter (optional)
2–3 drops lavender or rose oil

Place all the ingredients in a large glass bowl or resealable plastic bag. Gently mix by stirring or massaging the bag. Pour the powder into a clean cardboard box. To use: Sprinkle the powder on clean skin or apply with a powder puff.

Garden Note: Let your children write their names or a secret garden message with seeds and watch it grow! Simply choose a flat spot with good soil. With the end of a small stick or rake write your name, word, or message in the dirt. Plant seeds inside this line and cover them with more soil. Water well, and in a few weeks sprouts should appear. Good seeds to plant in this fashion are radishes, carrots, marigolds, and zinnias.

Yield: 8 ounces

Hundred Acre Wood Bath

1 cup water
½ cup honey
½ cup mild liquid soap

A. A. Milne's classic Pooh books are wonderful stories to read to young children. Everyone loves Winnie the Pooh, Christopher Robin's cuddly, stuffed toy bear. He lived with his friends in the Hundred Acre Woods and had a passion for "hunny" (honey). This foaming bath recipe contains Winnie's sweet passion and is perfect for soothing dry, sensitive skin.

Mix together all the ingredients and pour into a clean bottle with a tight-fitting stopper or lid. To use: Gently shake the bottle to reblend and pour ¼ cup into the bath under the running water.

Yield: 16 ounces, enough for eight baths

Lauren and Marie's Cooking Bath

½ cup mild liquid soap or baby wash
2 tablespoons fruit-flavored gelatin
½ cup water

My two daughters love to take "cooking baths." First we mix up a batch of this fruity bubble bath recipe. Then we gather up a collection of plastic cups, bowls, spoons, and funnels that may be used in the bath. They stir, pour, and mix themselves clean until I finally make them get out. We like to use fruit-flavored gelatin in this recipe as it gives the bathwater a fun color and scent. You may also substitute unflavored gelatin if you wish.

Mix together all ingredients and stir well until the gelatin has softened. To use: Pour the entire mixture under the running water as you fill the tub. Note: This bath may be mixed ahead of time and stored in a clean plastic jar or bottle.

Yield: 8 ounces, enough for one bath

ANIMAL TOPIARIES

My daughters and I made a wonderful fat rabbit for their garden and covered it with ivy. The girls love to place baskets of flowers in his outstretched paws. It was really rather simple to do. We made our own form using chicken wire, but you can also purchase topiary forms at many garden shops. We made a round body with a separate head and paws. This made moving our rabbit a bit easier. We covered the wire forms with sphagnum moss, securing it with plastic fishing line. We filled our form with good quality potting soil and then planted it with ivy. We made holes through the moss with sticks and stuffed the ivy through the holes in the chicken wire. We secured his head and paws onto the planted body with long, bamboo skewers. We gave him a good soaking and now water him about once a week.

Here are a few more tips my daughters and I learned about making animal topiaries:

- Simple shapes work best.

- Prune your shape often—they grow quickly and it is easy to end up with a big, green mound. Secure loose ends with floral pins or pieces of curved wire.

- Use sharp cutting shears. Dull blades can tear leaves and branches, resulting in brown areas.

- Two good plants to use are ivy and creeping fig. You can plant accent flowers for necklaces or clothes using seeds. Climbing snapdragon, nasturtium, and alyssum will quickly cover your shape.

- Have fun with your topiary by adding garden tools, baskets of flowers, hats and bows.

Alphabet Soap

2 cups gentle soap flakes (like
    grated Ivory Soap)
¼ to ½ cup water
A few drops food coloring
    (optional)
A few drops scented oils or extracts
    (optional)

This recipe makes a soapy dough that can be shaped into different letters of the alphabet for special bath-time words, names, and messages. You can also make simple shapes, such as hearts, squares, and balls. When it is time to wash up—after playing in the garden—these scented soaps are fun to use. They produce lots of bubbly water that will delight any child. You can also scent your soap shapes with oils and extracts.

Mix the soap flakes and water together until you have a smooth paste. You can do this by hand or use an electric mixer for a lighter, fluffier soap dough. You may need to increase the water or soap until you have a smooth mixture. Add a few drops of food coloring if you wish to color your soap mixture. Then blend in a few drops of scented oil and mix well. Lightly coat your hands with some cooking oil and mold the soap mixture into a letter or shape. Place the soap on a sheet of waxed paper and let it harden for several hours. To use: Enjoy as you would any bar of soap in the tub, shower, or next to the sink.

Yield: 12 ounces, 4 average-size soaps or 8 small soap letters

Peter Rabbit's Bath

We are all familiar with Beatrix Potter's tale of naughty Peter Rabbit who just could not keep out of Mr. MacGregor's garden. At the end of the tale Peter's mom gives him a cup of chamomile tea and sends him to bed. She is truly a wise mother as a good night's rest was just what her little bunny needed. Make up a batch of this chamomile bath for your own little ones. After the bath let them snuggle into their bed while you read them a bedtime story.

½ cup dried chamomile flowers
2 cups oatmeal
¼ cup cornstarch

Place all the ingredients inside a food processor or blender. Grind until you have a smooth, fine powder. The powder should have the consistency of whole-grain flour. Pour into a clean, airtight container or use a resealable plastic bag. To use: Pour ½ cup into your bath as you fill the tub or place inside muslin bags and hang under the flowing water faucet.

Garden Note: Decorate the tops of your garden stakes with colored marbles, pretty rocks, or small plastic figures. Use a good waterproof adhesive and your plants will have a fun support to climb up.

Yield: 16 ounces, enough for four baths

Garden Fairy Bath

1 tablespoon fresh thyme flowers
2 tablespoons assorted edible flower
    petals and leaves
½ cup nonfat dry milk
2 tablespoons grated mild soap

A bed of thyme was once thought to be the home of garden fairies. Old-time gardeners used to set aside small patches of this fragrant herb for the little magical beings to live among, because it was believed to be good luck to have a fairy in your garden. These small creatures would wear flower petal clothes and dine on small garden berries and leaves. They would only appear when the garden was silent and helped earn their way by keeping the plants neat and healthy. Fact or fancy? Just in case it's all true, I have a small patch of creeping thyme in a far corner of my yard. Treat your children to their own fantasy bath and let them imagine life among the tiny thyme flowers.

In a medium-size bowl mix together all the ingredients and stir well. To use: Pour the entire bath mixture under running water as you fill the tub.

Yield: 8 ounces, enough for one bath

Afternoon Face Paint

1 teaspoon cornstarch
1 teaspoon water
½ teaspoon cold cream (see page
    77 for recipe)
1–2 drops food coloring

*C*hildren love to imagine they are woodland fairies and garden elves, when they are dressed in daisy chains, flower garlands, and leaf hats. They can also paint their faces with colorful designs. With a little color and some imagination a boring afternoon suddenly becomes an exciting and imaginative day of fun and creativity! I use food coloring from the grocery store for the color, but you may also experiment with fresh berry juices and plant dyes to tint your face paints—just be sure they are safe for cosmetic use. You will need to mix up a batch for each color or double the recipe and divide it into small bowls before adding your dye.

Mix together the cornstarch, water, and cold cream and stir well until smooth. Add the food coloring one drop at a time and mix well until you are pleased with the shade. Spoon into a small jar or bowl. I have found reusable plastic paint palettes from art stores are good containers for your homemade paints. To use: Paint the skin using a small brush, cotton swab, or a clean finger-tip in any design you fancy. Clean off your designs with more cold cream and warm water.

Yield: ½ ounce

Flower Crowns

Growing up I spent many an afternoon sitting on our family lawn making daisy chains to wear as crowns and necklaces. Today my daughters and their friends enjoy this floral craft. They use all sorts of garden flowers, with the only requirement being they have strong, sturdy stems. To make your crown you will need a pair of scissors, a small knife, and a few paper clips.

24 fresh flowers with stems attached

Cut each flower stem to approximately three inches in length. Make a slit through the middle of each stem. To do this, lay the flower on a flat surface. Gently push the tip of the knife through the middle of the stem. To build your crown you will be making a chain. Pass one flower stem through the slit of another. Pulling the stems all the way through, keep passing flower stems through each other until you have a chain long enough to go around your head. To make the chain into a crown, use a paper clip to attach the last stem to the stem of the first flower.

Garden Note: Pioneer girls also made flower crowns. At night they would put them under their pillows to help them dream about their future.

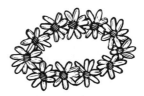

Yield: 1 flower crown

Sun Perfume

2 cups distilled water
1 crushed vitamin C tablet
1–2 large handfuls of fresh herb
    leaves and flower petals, washed
Assorted spices (optional)

This is a fun, scented project for young children to make. I call it Sun Perfume because the warm rays of the sun help release the aromatic oils from the fresh ingredients that scent your perfume. Let children pick their own combinations of fresh herbs and flowers and experiment with the scents they produce. They may also add a few dry spices, such as cinnamon sticks, anise stars, cardamom pods, or allspice berries to their mixtures. For stronger scents you can add a drop or two of essential oil to the finished perfumes.

Pour the water into a clean jar. Dissolve the vitamin C tablet in the water and stir well. Add your flowers, herbs, and spices. Place a lid or stopper on your jar and set it in a sunny spot indoors or outside in the garden. Gently shake your jar daily. After 3 days strain and discard the flowers and leaves, saving the scented water. Test the scent of your perfume by smelling it—for a stronger scent add more fresh ingredients and let the water sit for another 3 days. When you are satisfied with the scent of your perfume, pour it into a pretty bottle and enjoy!

Garden Note: In the summer when you water your lawn and garden, run through the sprinklers with your children!

Yield: 12–16 ounces

Scented Play Dough

Mix up a batch of this scented dough to have on hand when the kids need a quiet activity or you have children visiting. I like to use lavender oil to scent my dough, but other safe scents to use would be rose, vanilla, orange, peach, or coconut. Working and molding the scented mixture is a creative and calming activity. Let the children go out into the garden and gather some scented leaves and flower petals to knead into or decorate their creations. This recipe also makes a fun birthday gift for a special child—fill a bright pail with cookie cutters, funky kitchen gadgets, a small rolling pin, and a batch of scented play dough!

1 cup flour

½ cup salt

1 cup water (may be tinted with food coloring)

1 tablespoon sunflower oil

2 teaspoons cream of tartar

2–3 drops scented oil

2 tablespoons scented herb leaves or flower petals

Mix together the flour, salt, water, oil, and cream of tartar in a medium-size saucepan. Cook the mixture over medium heat until it begins to bubble. Remove the pan from the heat and stir in the scented oil and leaves and petals. Place the dough on a lightly floured board and knead for 3–5 minutes until smooth. Store in an airtight container. To use: Shape your dough into anything you desire. You can decorate it with small twigs, flowers, dried herbs, and spices. Store any leftover dough in a clean airtight container or resealable plastic bag. If left uncovered and allowed to air-dry your designs will dry out and harden.

Yield: **8 ounces**

Lavender Wands

Odd number of lavender stems
   (I like to use 13)
2 yards ⅜″-wide ribbon
Safety pin (optional)

Handmade lavender wands, or as the French call them *bouteilles* (bottles), are an easy herbal craft to teach children and one they can easily master. They will keep your drawers and closets smelling sweet and make lovely gifts for grandmothers, aunts, and neighbors. It is important to use freshly picked lavender as it is more pliable and easier to work with for small hands. Also, cut the stems as long as possible.

Gather your lavender stalks and tie them together tightly just under the flowers. Turn your bundle so that the flower heads are facing you. Gently, bend a stem at a time over the flower heads; repeat until all of the stalks are covering the flowers. You are making a sort of "basket" around the blooms to contain them after they dry. Start weaving your ribbon through the stalks, over and under. Continue weaving until you have covered all of the flowers. Wrap the ribbon tightly at the base of your weaving. Take a bit more ribbon and tie a bow at the base. Cut the stalks evenly to your desired wand length; you may also tie a bow around these ends. For small children you may want to attach a safety pin to the end of the ribbon to hold on to and make the weaving a bit easier. To use: Place the lavender next to the bed or in a drawer or closet. To refresh the scent, gently squeeze the woven end.

   Note: An even easier lavender wand can be made by simply bending back the stalks over the flower heads and tying—no weaving.

Yield: 1 lavender wand

Apricot Baby Oil

This is a light oil perfect for keeping young skin healthy and full of moisture. It is best used as a massage oil or after-bath lotion. Apricot kernel oil is made from the oil-rich nut inside the fruit's seed or pit. It is easily found at the grocery store in the cooking oil section. I like to make this recipe unscented, but if you prefer a subtle fragrance I would suggest using the mild essential oil of sweet orange, chamomile, or lavender—but only a drop or two.

¼ cup apricot kernel oil
1 tablespoon light sesame oil
½ tablespoon wheat germ oil
1–2 drops essential oil of sweet orange, chamomile, or lavender (optional)

Stir together all ingredients and pour into a clean, dry container with a tight-fitting lid. To use: Massage a small amount into warm or damp skin. Store in a cool, dark, dry location.

Garden Note: Use plant markers and label your herbs and flowers for your children. Even better, let them make the small signs. This is a great way for them to learn the names of all their favorite plants.

Yield: 3 ounces

MASSAGING BABIES

In recent years the ancient art of baby massage has gained renewed interest. Once regarded as an essential skill of motherhood passed down from mother to daughter, this activity had been all but lost in our society until recently. There are now classes for new mothers, books, and even videos on the art of baby massage. It is believed that by gently massaging your baby's body, he/she will grow stronger, sleep better, eat more, and even gain relief from colic. It also encourages bonding and acts as a form of communication between new parents and their baby.

(continued)

Because babies are so new to the world and their sense of smell is extremely sensitive, I would not use a scented oil when massaging a baby under twelve months of age. Pure, sweet almond oil works well and is gentle enough for a newborn.

I used to massage my babies after bathing them and before putting them to bed at night. You should choose a time that is relaxing and enjoyable for both of you. Here are the basic steps I followed:

1. Sit with your baby on your lap or place your baby on a soft mat in front of you. It is important that you are both in a comfortable position.

2. With your baby facing you, place your hands on his/her hips, and slide your hand up to the shoulders then down the sides of his/her body. Repeat several times.

3. Massage your baby's stomach, gently stroking it in a circular motion.

4. Stroke the back of your baby's hands and then the palms. Gently squeeze each finger and repeat with the other hand.

5. Massage the arms. Holding his/her hand in yours, stroke in a flowing motion from the shoulder to the wrist.

6. Massage the legs. Hold his/her foot in your hand and stroke each leg from the thigh to the ankle. Repeat several times. Squeeze and rotate each toe and massage the foot.

7. Turn your baby over and massage the back of the body. Use calm, gentle strokes. Slow, light strokes are very soothing to your baby.

You and your baby will soon be looking forward to this special time of comfort and relaxation. Enjoy!

Coco Crazy Body Oil

*O*ne whiff of this rich tropical oil and my daughters named it Coco Crazy. Coconut palms have always been one of our favorite trees. They are tall, graceful, and produce coconuts! Dried coconut meat is called copra and is where coconut oil originates. It is used to make fragrant skin and hair oils and is also mild and gentle enough for young skin. The word coco is Spanish for a grinning face; this coco refers to the three dots or eyes on the fruit's base that look like a funny mask. It may also apply to your children's laughs and giggles as they apply this rich, tropical body oil.

2 tablespoons coconut oil
½ tablespoon grated cocoa butter
2 tablespoons castor oil
2 drops coconut fragrance oil
   (optional)

In a heat-resistant container mix together the coconut oil, cocoa butter, and castor oil. Heat gently in the microwave or in a water bath until the coconut oil and cocoa butter are melted. Stir well and add the coconut fragrance for a stronger scent. Let the mixture cool completely then pour into a clean bottle. To use: Massage a small amount into warm skin after bathing.

Garden Note: The garden is the perfect place to read to your child.

Yield: 2 ounces

Diaper
Cream

2 tablespoons soy lecithin
1 teaspoon coconut oil
1 teaspoon apricot kernel oil
¼ teaspoon vitamin E oil
½ cup distilled water

Today, with the use of washing machines and disposable diapers, diaper rash is no longer the common baby rash it once was. Babies' bottoms are kept drier and they are getting changed more often. This keeps their delicate skin dry and comfortable and gives it a chance to breathe. If your little one's delicate bum does happen to break out, this old-fashioned cure has stood the test of time. It contains liquid lecithin, a substance extracted from soybeans and used for ages as an excellent moisturizer and diaper ointment. It protects baby's sensitive skin and keeps it dry. It should be applied once a day. For extreme cases, use this cream every time you change your baby's diaper.

Mix together the lecithin, coconut oil, apricot kernel oil, and vitamin E oil. Heat this mixture gently until the coconut oil is liquefied. Gently heat the distilled water until it is roughly the same temperature as the oil mixture. Pour the lecithin mixture into a blender and start stirring. Slowly add the warm water and blend on High until the mixture is thick and creamy. Pour the cream into a clean container and allow it to cool completely, stirring occasionally. To use: Apply a small amount onto your baby's clean bottom before diapering.

Note: You can adjust this cream's consistency by adding more or less water to the recipe.

Yield: 6 ounces

HOME SWEET SUNFLOWER HOME

It is easy to plant your own secret garden clubhouse by planting sunflowers in a circular pattern. These giant garden flowers will become the walls of your house. Climbing plants and flowers, such as morning glories, loofah sponges, cucumbers, and beans can be planted under the sunflowers. They will use the giant flower stalks as climbing poles and natural supports. Their leaves and greenery will help fill in your walls. You may also cover the ground inside your house with a fragrant carpet of creeping herbs such as mint, chamomile, or thyme. No house would be complete without plenty of fresh flowers, so make sure to plant a few bright zinnias, marigolds, and cosmos next to the doorway. No roof is needed on your home; sitting inside and gazing up at the huge flower heads and sunny sky above is what this house is all about!

All the plants I have mentioned are easy to grow from seeds. Given a good soil base, and plenty of sunlight and water, your house should be complete in 60–75 days. Of course, you can move in right away and let your home grow around you.

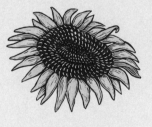

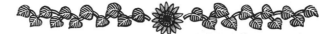

Glossary

Acid: Liquid, solid, or gas that contains hydrogen and reacts with metals to form salts and water. You can usually tell an acid by its pH level, which is below 7. Examples of common acids are citric acid (lemon juice), malic acid (apples), acetic acid (vinegar), and tannic acid (found in tea).

Acid mantle: Microscopic film of acidic moisture over the skin; a kind of protective covering.

Alcohol: A colorless, volatile liquid obtained by distillation and fermentation of carbohydrates (grain, molasses, potatoes). Alcohol is antiseptic and cooling but is also very drying to the hair and skin; care should thus be taken not to use too much.

Antiseptic: A substance that stops the growth of bacteria and helps to control infection by inhibiting germs.

Astringent: A product that makes the skin feel refreshed. It may also give a tightened sensation to the skin as the ingredients evaporate. Usually recommended for oily skin types as astringents can be drying to the skin and hair.

Combination skin: Both dry and oily areas; the most common skin type.

Compost: Mixture of decaying organic matter, such as leaves, grass clippings, and fruit peels, used as a soil additive and fertilizer.

Cosmetics: Defined by the Federal Drug Act in 1938 as (1) articles intended to be rubbed, poured, sprinkled, or sprayed on, introduced into, or otherwise applied to the human body or any part thereof for cleansing, beautifying, promoting attractiveness, or altering the appearance; and (2) articles intended for use as a component of any such articles.

Dermis: Inner layer of the skin, protected by the epidermis, and made up of tissues, muscles, and nerves. Collagen is found in the dermis layer.

Dry skin: Description of skin that feels tight after washing and has a tendency to flake; the pores are small and the skin is thin.

Emollient: A thick, creamy material used to soothe or soften the skin. Emollients are usually made from oil, water, and wax. A classic emollient is basic cold cream.

Emulsifier: A material that binds two different materials together. An example of this would be beeswax, used in creams to bind together the oil and water and keep them from separating.

Epidermis: The surface layer of the skin. The epidermis is where new cells are constantly being formed.

Exfoliation: Removal of dead skin cells and surface dirt, a very important step in proper skin care because removing dead skin cells allows the skin to function more efficiently and to absorb more moisture.

Facial: A total treatment for the face that consists of deep-cleansing, conditioning, and moisturizing the skin.

Fuller's earth: A fine gray clay powder that comes from algae found in seabeds and riverbeds and is particularly high in magnesium silicate. The name comes from the clay's use in making woolen fabrics—"fulling" was a way of increasing the weight and bulk of the cloth by shrinking and beating it; a fuller was the person who made the woolen material.

Herb: A plant or plant part valued for its medicinal, savory, or aromatic qualities. For example, chamomile is very soothing to the skin, peppermint has a scent that is extremely refreshing, and geranium oil kills bacteria.

Humectant: A substance that holds the moisture in a product or on the skin. Honey is a wonderful natural humectant. Glycerine is the most popular humectant used in cosmetic products.

Infusion: A mixture of herbs and water that are soaked together for a period of time. When you make tea, you are making an infusion.

Kaolin clay: Sometimes called China clay, this is a fine white powder originally obtained from Kaolin Hill in Kiangsi Province in southeast China. Kaolin clay is rich in aluminum silicate. It can be purchased at natural food stores and pharmacies.

Natural: A term loosely used, and no one seems to agree on its definition with regard to cosmetics. The Food and Drug Administration is currently trying to come up with an official definition. I think of natural as not containing any manmade ingredients. Natural to me means "as found in nature." Some feel that natural means no chemicals, but chemicals are natural. Everything in our world is made up of chemical elements.

Normal skin: Clear, firm skin with few blemishes; not dry or oily.

Occlusive oil: A substance that increases the water content of the skin by creating a seal on the surface, holding in moisture. Canola, olive, sesame, and castor oil are all examples of occlusive oils.

Oily skin: Description of skin that feels a little greasy and has a shine that does not go away, enlarged pores, and no lines.

Organic: A substance that is or once was living. In chemistry, organic means "containing a carbon atom."

pH: The measure of acidity and alkalinity in a solution. The pH scale goes from 0–14 (neutral is 7). Healthy skin may range from pH 3 to 5½.

Ultraviolet light: The invisible light rays that penetrate the epidermis and have been proven to cause premature aging and skin cancer.

U.S.P.: Stands for United States Pharmacopeia and means that the product meets the standards for use set by the United States Pharmaceutical Board. You will see this labeling on many products, such as lanolin, camphor, glycerine, and alum powder.

Water Bath: This is a method for indirectly heating ingredients when making cosmetics. A heat-resistant container (like a glass jar) containing ingredients is placed in a shallow pan with 1–2 inches of water. The water is heated over medium heat, melting the ingredients inside the jar. It's similar to a double boiler in function because the ingredients are protected from direct heat. Also known as a bain marie. The water bath can also be made using an electric skillet filled with 1–2 inches of water.

Index

exfoliants/exfoliation, 21, 73, 151,
      168, 215, 218, 230
exotic fragrances, 258
Extreme Soak, 201
eye dropper, 11
eyebright, 108
eyes, tired, 108, 109

face paints, 294–95
facial(s), 76–77
facial care products/treatments,
      71–114
facial masks, 8, 17, 74, 75, 77,
      96–108
   anise in, 89
   peach, 51
facial scrubs, 84–85, 113
facial steams, 112–13, 186
farmers' markets, 5, 18, 19
fat
   in soap, 159, 160, 161
fennel, 79, 98, 113, 122
fennel leaves, 125
fennel seeds, 89
fern leaves, 153
Feverfew Complexion Milk, 82
feverfew leaves, 82
flax, 66, 122
flaxseed, 39, 66
Fleur-de-Lis Body Powder,
      271–72
Floral Facial Steam, 111–12
floral fragrances, 258
floral hat band, 5, 62
Flower Crowns, 285, 295
flower meditation, 249
flower petals, 26
   in bath products, 192, 193, 203
   facial steam, 112–13
Flower Power Bath, 193
flowering tree branches, forcing,
      55
flowers
   drying, 28
   in garden clubhouse, 303
   labeling, 299

language of, 206–7
pressing, 64
scents, 281
in soap, 163
foaming bath salts, 203
food dehydrator, 25, 26, 28
foot care products, 133, 134,
      146–55
foot creams, 133, 154
foot mask, 146, 153
foot massage, 146, 147, 151, 236
Foot Odor Cure, 154–55
foot powder, 134, 154
foot soaks, 134
footbaths, 133, 134, 148–52
   herbs for, 150
Four Seasons Facial, 76–77
fragrance
   basic scent groups, 258
   mystique surrounding, 258
fragrance garden, 259, 280–81
fragrance products, 255–81
frangipani, 247
frangipani trees, 247
freezing, 25, 28, 127
French green clay, 107
Fresh Carrot Mask, 102–3
fresh flower arrangements, 137
Fresh Gingerroot Bath, 191
Fresh Mowed Grass, 263–64
Fresh Peppermint Toothpaste,
      118, 128
Fresh Spearmint Lip Gloss, 124
Fresh-as-a-Daisy Soap, 167
frizzy hair, 65
frost, protecting plants from, 122
fruit fragrances, 258, 263
fruit trees, 102
Fuller's earth, 107
funnel, 11

Galen's Cold Cream, 77–78
Gallica Rose Bath, 190
garden(s), 25
   bath herbs and flowers in, 174
   children's, 286, 289

colonial, 267
fragrance, 280–81
fragrant leaves and petals in, 259
healthy complexion, 113–14
healthy skin care, 231
Japanese-style, 196
literary, 285
natural beauty from, 3–6
peace of mind, 252
place to read, 301
relaxation in, 235, 237
zodiac, 177
garden bath, 208
garden beauty party, 214
Garden Boot Bath, 149
garden clubhouse, 303
Garden Fairy Bath, 294
garden party, 213
garden pests, 50, 51, 95
garden scents, 257
garden teas, 180
garden tools, 33
   cleaning, 195
gardener's gift basket, 155
gardenias, 179, 281
gardening, 4
   container, 31–32
   and relaxation, 235
   using cold cream in, 78
gardening basics, 29–34
gardening projects for children,
      286
garden-stained hands, 145
gelatin, 290
geranium, 88, 231
   scented, 57, 89, 90, 273
   in skin care, 73
geranium leaves, 90
Geranium Petal Body Scrub,
      219–20
geranium rose oil, 89
German Chamomile Tea Soother,
      95
gifts
   bath products, 174, 176, 177,
      184, 185, 189, 192, 205

Poison Ivy, 222
pomanders, scented, 274–75
poppies, 5, 110
potassium, 18, 20, 21, 97
potato cleanser, 81
Potato Mask, 96
potatoes, 50–51, 73, 231
potpourri, 5, 199, 258–59, 276–79
    bath, 206–7
    personal, 279
pots, 31–32
    decorating, 57
Prehistoric Nail Strengthener,
    138
preservation, 23–28
    herbs, 40
preservatives, 8, 22
pressed-flower combs and
    brushes, 64, 69
Pretty Polly Geranium Rinse, 57
protein, 104, 133
pumice powder, 151
pumice stone, 146, 149, 152, 155
pumpkins, 220
purple coneflower (echinacea),
    185

quality control, 9
quince seeds, 39

radishes, 103, 289
rainwater, 111
raspberries, 127
Raspberry Chocolate Mint
    Mouthwash, 127
raspberry leaves
    hair rinse, 56
Ray's Relaxation Blend, 247
recipes, 5, 7–9
red clover, 121
Red Clover Lip Gel, 119, 121
reflexology, 147
Refreshing Eye Gel, 109
refrigeration, 8, 39, 119, 213
relaxation, 233–53, 261
Rhassoul mud, 107

Rhubarb Hair Lightener, 60
rhubarb plants, 60
rhubarb stalk, 271
rice flour, 272
rinses
    face, 77
    hair, 38–39, 41, 50–51, 53–58,
        59, 69
River Stone Footbath, 150–51
rock collection, 242
rock salt, 202
Roman Fennel Mask, 98
rosa rugosa, 107
rose (scent), 258, 261, 281
Rose Geranium Splash, 89–90
rose hips, 106, 107
rose oil, 297
rose petals, 27, 112, 125
    in bath products, 178
    in fragrance products, 260
    in lip glosses, 119
rose spice
    in soap, 163
rosemary, 28, 122
    growing indoors, 99
    in hair care products, 38, 39,
        45, 57, 69
    in massage oils, 247
    memory-enhancing, 98, 99
    in skin care products, 98–99,
        112
rosemary (scent), 258, 280
Rosemary Conditioner, 48–49
rosemary oil, 46
rosemary plants, 49
roses, 231
    in bath products, 187, 190, 193
    black spot/mildew on, 240
    in massage oils, 240
    tips for cutting, 43
    watering, 260
rosewater, 20, 260
    as deodorant, 226
    shampoo, 43
    in skin care products, 77, 80,
        93, 106

rubber gloves, 143–44, 161
rum, 18

sachets, 192, 259, 277–78
"Safe Sun," 75
sage, 28, 122, 129
    in hair care products, 38, 39,
        45, 53, 69
    in skin care products, 99, 112
sage (scent), 280
sage leaves, 125
sage plants, 53
Sage Tea Rinse, 53
Saint-John's-Wort Oil, 245
salicylic acid, 100
salt, 21
salt rubs, 218
sand, beach, 146
sandalwood, 20
sandalwood (scent), 258
saponification, 160–61, 163
Saturn's Aftershave, 258, 266
scalp, 39, 52, 55, 56, 57
    Scented Massage Oil, 63
    Stimulating Scalp Toner, 40
scalp massage, 236
Scarborough Fair Shampoo, 45
scent groups, basic, 258
Scented Bath Pillow, 205
Scented Bath Sachets, 192
scented bath salts, 202, 205
Scented Play Dough, 286, 297
Scented Scalp Massage Oil, 39,
    63
Scented Sugar Scrubs, 85
scents, 8
    alcohol-free, 258
    creating, 257
    human responds to, 257, 280
    in meditation and massage, 236
    for solid perfume, 263
scrubs, 73–74
    body, 212, 219–20
    facial, 84–85, 113
sea salt, 150, 177
sebum, 86